The Stroke Book

THE STROKE BOOK

One-on-One Advice About Stroke Prevention, Management, and Rehabilitation

Arthur Ancowitz, M.D.

William Morrow and Company, Inc.
New York

This book is based on current medical research, knowledge, and understanding, and to the best of the author's and editors' ability, the material is accurate and valid. Even so, any individual reader should not use the information to alter a prescribed regimen or in any form of self-treatment without first seeking the advice of his or her personal physician. The author and editors do not bear any responsibility or liability for the information or for any uses to which it may be put. The information contained in this book is not intended as a substitute for appropriate medical treatment.

Library of Congress Cataloging-in-Publication Data

Ancowitz, Arthur, 1925–
    The stroke book : one-on-one advice about stroke prevention,
    management, and rehabilitation / by Arthur Ancowitz.
        p.   cm.
    Includes bibliographical references and index.
    ISBN 0-688-09055-9
    1. Cerebrovascular disease—Popular works. 2. Cerebrovascular
    disease—Prevention. 3. Cerebrovascular disease—Patients—
    Rehabilitation. I. Title.
    RC388.5.A5   1993
    616.8'1—dc20   92-27999
                                                                CIP

Printed in the United States of America

First Edition

1 2 3 4 5 6 7 8 9 10

BOOK DESIGN BY ARLENE SCHLEIFER GOLDBERG
LINE ART © 1993 BY JUDY STAGNITTO

Preface

The beauty of an unfettered brain—a brain that can express love, sense the seasons, smell the fragrances, feel the joys of life, experience sweet memories—is that it holds tremendous promise, tremendous capacity to enhance our lives.

Injured, however, the brain leaves us with sorrows and a deep sense of inadequacy. Reason, mood, behavior, movement, and feelings fall hostage to damage, denial, and even death.

That's the tragedy that often follows a stroke. Just imagine a person who is frustrated because he or she cannot move a limb in response to an inner wish. Or imagine the reaction of one who is close to such a victim of brain damage. Now, multiply by two million, and you have an idea of the magnitude of the tragedy, for that's the number of people who now suffer from stroke impairment in the United States.

How can you measure this sadness and the sadness of family members and friends of the victims? Such sadness can't be quantified; it can only be felt. Yet the *ultimate* sadness is that so many strokes could have been prevented—and that brings me to a major purpose of this book.

In dealing with the prevention, management, and rehabilitation of stroke over the years, both as a practicing physician and as the director of the Stroke Foundation, Inc., I've developed something close to a crusader mentality: I know what's *possible* for stroke victims as well as for those at risk for stroke. Yet despite the promise of help and good health, the reality falls short of the promise. Too many still fall prey to the ravages of stroke because the general public remains woefully uninformed.

In the following pages, I'll do whatever I can to elevate the general level of knowledge and provide the information necessary to enable us to respond successfully to stroke. Together, you and I will explore ways to bring the latest medical advances to bear on the needs of the average person. I am indebted to my patients who taught me so much.

In preparing this book, I'm grateful to Bill Adler for suggesting such a book and for introducing me to William Proctor, a skilled writer who has been helpful in the creation of this book; my editor at William Morrow and Company, Randy Ladenheim-Gil and her assistant, Steve Wilson, for their patience and encouragement; chief librarian Shirley E. Dansker, assistant librarian Julia Chai, and library assistant Laura Stark of the Lenox Hill Hospital library.

I am also grateful for the friendship of and the direct and indirect assistance given to me by Dr. Arthur E. Schwartz, Dr. Joseph Cimino, Dr. Kasriel Eilender, Dr. Wayne Decker, Dr. Murray Goldstein, Dr. Valery Lanyi, Dr. Matthew Lee, Dr. Brian Reynolds, Dr. Albert Harary, Dr. Lawrence Kaplan, Dr. Jay Rosenblum, Dr. Steve Tucci, Dr. Thomas Raymond, Dr. Ron Lawrence, Dr. George Sheehan, Dr. Michael Bruno, Dr. Ira Hoffman, Dr. Angelo Taranta, Dr. Stanley Barasch, Dr. Fletcher H. McDowell, Dr. Peter Herman, Dr. Murray A. Grossman, Dr. Egon Fisher, Dr. Richard Orphanos, and Dr. Irina Gerasimova.

The basis for most advances in medicine is due to the researchers in the basic and clinical sciences. We all owe them a debt of gratitude and more financial assistance.

Dr. Michael B. Finklestein is gratefully acknowledged for his review of this manuscript.

I wish to thank Elizabeth Hazlett, Pearl Edwards, Marina

Gotay, and Edythe Lachlan for their assistance; and my family for their forbearance and support.

Finally, a word about the Stroke Foundation, Inc., which tries to help stoke victims and their families by answering their questions.

The Stroke Foundation was chartered in the state of New York in 1967. It was founded by a group of friends whose relatives had suffered strokes. The late Saul Davis and his wife, Vivian Davis, acted as attorneys pro bono in setting up the organization. The basic purpose was to disseminate information about stroke.

The foundation laid the groundwork for the issue of two other publications: *Strokes and Their Prevention* in 1975 and *What You Should Know About Stroke Prevention* in 1979. The latter was sponsored by the U.S. Department of Health, Education and Welfare (NIH Publication No. 79-1909).

There are no paid officers or employees of the Stroke Foundation.

Volunteers have been the backbone of the Stroke Foundation. The late Alex Weinstein took care of the mechanics of receiving requests for information and asking me to reply when he could not. Since 1967, hundreds of letters and phone calls have been received annually from all over the country and from many foreign countries as well.

Contributions in the names of loved ones who have had strokes are acknowledged. No fund-raising activities have ever been held. The foundation is in need of funds and volunteers, particularly those with organizational experience and talents.

Contents

The Stroke Book

Chapter One

Let's Talk About Stroke

When the wife of Dr. Robert M., a leading New York physician, called me one Sunday afternoon, I could tell by the anxious tone of her voice that something was seriously wrong.

"Robert can't speak!" she said. "He's seeing his patients, but he can't talk to them!"

When I arrived at Bob's office, I was confronted by an amazing sight: Here was this energetic, highly successful, healthy-looking physician, working at the same pace on a Sunday as he did during the rest of the week, with a full staff rushing about to do his bidding—yet he couldn't say a word to them!

He was furiously jotting off notes, using hand signals with nurses and trying to communicate with his patients through his wife, who was acting as an "interpreter." Yet all the while, he was becoming more and more frustrated by his incapacity.

After a few minutes of questioning, I learned from notes, hand and head signals, and further explanations from his wife that Robert had been without speech for about an hour. He had suddenly lost his ability to talk. Also, he indicated that he was having some trouble seeing out of one eye; he was a little lightheaded; and overall, he felt weak on the left side of his body.

"Robert, you've had a stroke," I told him. "You know as well as I do that it's *essential* for you to act *quickly* if you're going to recover completely. Damage is still probably occurring in your brain, but luckily, we are at the very beginning of this thing, so we can limit the injury. I'm going to admit you to the hospital right now for further tests in preparation for treatment."

He seemed to protest mildly. But even though he had been trying to ignore or deny what was happening to him, now the cold light of reality was dawning.

After Bob entered the hospital, a series of tests were arranged, including a CAT scan and an arteriogram. The CAT, or CT (which is the acronym for "computed tomography"), involves the use of a computer and X rays to produce black-and-white pictures of slices of the brain. The arteriogram requires threading a very thin, flexible tube into the arteries and then injecting a dye into the blood through this tube. X-ray pictures taken of the dye-enhanced vessels can provide very clear pictures of the brain's arteries.

The CAT scan showed that there had been no hemorrhage in the brain. The arteriogram, on the other hand, revealed a partial obstruction of the carotid artery on the right side of his neck. A clot had lodged at a narrowing of the vessel at this spot and had reduced the flow of blood to the speech center of the brain. As a result, Robert had lost his ability to talk.

Without further delay, an anticlotting agent, heparin, was prescribed, and fortunately, Robert responded quite well. With a few days of medication and speech therapy, he regained much of his speaking capacity.

Because of the possibility of a future stroke owing to the obstruction in his neck, Robert was referred to a center experienced in the surgical treatment of cervical (neck) atherosclerosis. Eventually, he underwent a procedure involving the removal of a clot and fatty matter from the offending artery.

Today, Robert is conducting his medical practice as vigorously as ever and is proof that fast, effective action can often return a stroke victim to normal. Now on a low-fat, low-cholesterol diet (see Chapter Five), he also takes one aspirin daily and exercises moderately. Perhaps most important of all, he no longer needs speech therapy!

But things haven't always been this promising on the medical front.

———How Times Do Change———

In the past, stroke victims were generally regarded as lost causes by family members and physicians alike. Recovery from stroke was deemed even more unlikely than improvement after a heart attack. In fact, there was a heavy atmosphere of despair that was shared by patients, their family, and their physicians.

The paralysis, loss of speech, and other disabilities that accompany stroke resulted in patients who were regarded as slightly less than human objects, useless for normal daily tasks and good mainly for sitting around, waiting for the next stroke and death. The patients with stroke were often referred to as "vegetables" or "crocks" by those who should have known better.

Fortunately, this negative attitude toward stroke has changed. Now, there is more of a can-do mentality. In fact, stroke treatment *can* be accomplished effectively through a variety of sensible options. Here are some of the many encouraging breakthroughs that research and hard work have provided in recent years.

* Investigations are being conducted on new medications that can dissolve blood clots and otherwise improve the chances of recovery of stroke patients.

* Various surgical procedures can clear out obstructions in the blood vessels.

* Medications as simple as aspirin may help in stroke prevention. Other medications are available when aspirin can't be used.

* Improved neurosurgical techniques have been developed.

* The role of antioxidants and glutamate blockers has increased.

* Scans, including sound scans as well as CT and MRI (magnetic resonance imaging), are more accessible.

* Diets can be fine-tuned in order to head off the development of atherosclerosis (hardening of the arteries)—the principal cause of stroke.

* High blood pressure, a major cause of stroke, can almost always be controlled through medications.

* Rehabilitation has advanced far both as a science and as an art in helping stroke victims return to productivity.

All in all, these and other new developments have greatly reduced the "morbidity," or damage to the brain, caused by stroke. To appreciate the exciting medical advances—and what they can mean to you as a patient or potential patient— it will be helpful at this early point in our discussion to lay down a working definition of stroke.

What Is Stroke?

A stroke is a loss of functioning brain tissue, with an accompanying disability, such as muscle weakness, paralysis, blindness, or speech impairment. Strokes are triggered by a deprivation of blood to a part of the brain.

As the third leading cause of death in the United States, behind heart disease and cancer, stroke is expensive: The annual cost of medical care for the problem is enormous. It has been estimated to cost on the order of $25 billion per year.

Nearly 500,000 Americans suffer a stroke every year, and 150,000 die from the condition. Presently, 3 million people in the United States have survived a stroke, and many of them continue to live with some disability. Stroke is the leading cause of disabilities in our country.

What sort of circulatory disturbances may lead to a stroke? There are four causes, which we will discuss in some detail in Chapter 2. In the meantime, here they are in summary form:

Cause 1: a stationary clot. The process of atherosclerosis, or clogging of the arteries with fatty deposits, including cholesterol, can affect the brain as well as the heart. A buildup of fats in the arteries leading to the brain—as happened with Dr. Robert M. in our example above—will narrow those vessels until they become vulnerable to being almost completely closed off. A narrowed vessel is referred to as stenosis.

This stationary clot acts as a kind of plug, shutting off the flow of blood to a particular area of the brain, and a stroke results. The clot that stops the flow is known in medical parlance as a thrombus, and so doctors call this type of stroke a thrombotic stroke. The brain tissue that is deprived of blood and dies is said to be "infarcted." This type of condition accounts for almost two thirds of all strokes.

Cause 2: a traveling clot. A clot may also develop in the heart or blood vessels and travel through the circulatory system until it lodges at a particular site in or near the brain. There, it will plug the blood flow and cause a stroke, just as the stationary clot does. This type of traveling plug, which causes about 5–10 percent of strokes, is called an embolism or embolus, and the stroke is known as an embolic stroke.

Cause 3: a bleeding artery in the brain. A weakness may occur in the wall of an artery in the brain. Usually the cause is high blood pressure. This is called "essential" hypertension when the cause of high blood pressure is unknown. Eventually, the vessel may rupture, and the resulting bleeding or leakage—called a cerebral hemorrhage—will flood a small portion of the brain. This kind of attack occurs in almost 20 percent of all strokes.

Cause 4: a balloonlike weakness in one of the brain's blood vessels. Weakness in the wall of an artery can result in a balloonlike outcropping, which is called an aneurysm. It occurs in the lower part of the brain, known as the base of the brain.

Blood can break through a weak point in the aneurysm and spread into the fluid that surrounds the brain. This fluid is called the cerebrospinal fluid, or simply spinal fluid. The bleeding is known as subarachnoid bleeding or hemorrhage because it penetrates the membranes that cover the brain (one of which is called the arachnoid membrane).

Congenital malformation of arteries and veins in the brain, called arteriovenous malformation, can also cause bleeding into the spinal fluid. Subarachnoid hemorrhage occurs in 5 percent to 10 percent of all strokes. Young people participating in contact sports are among the most common victims of these types of strokes.

Aneurysms as well as A-V malformations are treatable through surgical correction. Speed and skilled care are urgent.

We'll be exploring these causes of stroke more extensively in the following chapter, but this brief description should at least give you a preliminary idea about what happens during a stroke. Before we go any further, however, let's dispel a few of the common myths.

Myths and Realities About Stroke

Myth 1: Strokes can't be prevented.

Reality: In fact, you *can* prevent strokes—by changing your diet, lowering blood pressure, and taking other aggressive steps to improve your health.

The preventability of stroke is supported by hard facts. During the decade 1975–86, the death rate from stroke declined a remarkable 33 percent, according to a 1988 report by the National Institute of Neurological and Communicative Disorders and Stroke.

While we don't know all the reasons for this decline, some are probably related to the prevention and survival strategies we'll be discussing in this book. Among other things, increasing numbers of people are learning how to lower or eliminate various risk factors, such as hypertension (sustained high blood pressure), obesity, high cholesterol, and nicotine addiction.

Myth 2: Middle-aged and younger people don't have to worry about strokes.

Reality: To the contrary, middle-aged and younger people may suffer a stroke if they have such conditions as high blood pressure. As we've already seen, ruptured aneurysms, while uncommon, do strike younger people. It *is* true that most strokes occur among people who are over sixty years of age, but younger people are by no means immune. The use of drugs such as cocaine has been implicated.

Myth 3: It's impossible to predict whether you're a candidate for stroke.

Reality: You will learn in this book how to evaluate your relative chances for stroke from the various risk factors described in Chapter Three. You'll also be taught how to identify and interpret preliminary signals that a stroke may be imminent.

These warning signals include the so-called transient ischemic attack, or TIA. A TIA is a kind of ministroke from which patients usually recover completely within about twenty-four hours. Most TIAs last between one and five minutes. Half of those who have a TIA and are not treated will have a stroke within one year. In general, those who suffer a major stroke may have first experienced a TIA.

Symptoms of the TIA are much the same as for a regular stroke—speech problems, muscle weakness, loss of sight, or mental confusion. An alert patient will notify his physician, who in turn will evaluate and take action. Anticlotting drugs or other medication to head off the onset of a full-fledged stroke are often prescribed.

Myth 4: You can never recover significantly from a stroke.

Reality: Wrong again! In fact, only 15 percent of those who have had a stroke become significantly incapacitated, with such disabilities as permanent loss of speech or of the ability to walk. Two thirds of the nearly half million people who have a stroke each year survive, and one third recover sufficiently to go back to their normal activities. About one half may continue to have some handicap, such as a speech impediment or partial paralysis. But many of those patients recover to a large extent with proper therapy and medications.

Myth 5: One stroke will almost always lead to a second.

Reality: It is true that for those who have had one stroke, the chances are greater that they'll experience a second one.

But in many cases, the second attack can be prevented with medications and life-style changes. Strategies to prevent the second stroke will be discussed in the survival plan presented in Chapter Six.

The facts already discussed suggest strongly that stroke *can* be prevented or the effects can be minimized by those who develop a sound survival strategy.

Your Personal Plan— _____and Our Partnership_____

Throughout this book, I will be giving you information and advice and exhorting you to do what you need to do to prevent stroke, to recover from stroke, or to lower your risk. Obviously, I can't actually serve as your personal physician, and I wouldn't want to try! Your own physician is your best resource, and you should discuss any questions you have with him or her. But I do want to provide you with information that will allow you to observe, understand, and communicate more intelligently with your *real* physician. To this end, here is a sampling of some of the topics we will be discussing:

* The symptoms that signal the onset of a stroke—and the events that begin to occur in the brain when blood flow is reduced or cut off

* The "rules of risk"—including the relative threats from such factors as age, hypertension, diabetes, blood fat imbalances, obesity, smoking, and contraceptives

* Ways the reader can reduce his or her risk of stroke

* How to meet hypertension head-on through medications and life-style changes

* The most powerful attack on artery disease—guidelines for preventing atherosclerosis, or clogging of the arteries leading to the brain

* Why prevention of a *second* stroke is so important in first-stroke therapy

* "Cutting edge" medications such as TPA, which is currently being studied in many medical centers

* Surgical treatments for the prevention of stroke

* Diagnostic procedures, such as computed tomography (CT), positron emission tomography (PET), single-photon emission computed tomography (SPECT), and magnetic resonance imaging (MRI)

* Techniques for rehabilitating the stroke victim

Finally, the book concludes with a section in which the most common questions about stroke are answered. There, I'll deal with such frequently asked questions as these:

Is there a stroke personality?

What about the benefits of diet?

Can I really expect full recovery?

How can I quit smoking?

What are the chances I'll have a stroke if one of my parents had one?

To sum up, then, we are about to embark on a medical adventure that should significantly increase the chances that you or your loved ones will live longer, more productive lives. Our first stop on this survival expedition will be the heart—or to be more precise, the head—of the matter: the symptoms and physical responses that occur when stroke strikes.

Chapter Two

What Happens When Stroke Strikes?

The threat of stroke triggers tremendous fears because the very center of our intelligence and personal identity, the brain, is the target of the attack.

While the term "brain attack" may seem unsophisticated, Dr. Vladimir Hachinski, a leading stroke expert from the University of Western Ontario, has suggested that this term best describes stroke. So, just as a "heart attack" is associated with the attitude "Get yourself to the emergency room!" a "brain attack" or stroke should be identified with getting medical advice and assistance immediately. The reason: Techniques for responding to both these crises have greatly improved in recent years, but to be maximally effective, they need to be applied *as soon as possible* after the attack begins.

The traditional medical term for a stroke, "cerebrovascular accident" (CVA), means literally a damaging event in the blood vessels in the brain that is beyond one's control. But "CVA" doesn't tell the story as accurately as do the terms "brain attack" and "stroke." Those last two terms convey more of a sense of urgency and demand an immediate response.

We become concerned about stroke not just because death may occur, but also because there may be serious deterioration of mental functioning. Some people may feel a temporary surge of anxiety or fear when they are confronted with a blow-by-blow description of the damage inflicted by a stroke. But I'm willing to take that risk for two reasons: First, I am a great believer that the more information and knowledge you have, the better able you are to cope with worries and crises—including medical worries and crises. Second, I'm convinced that an understanding of the mechanisms of stroke will motivate more people to act quickly if the brain comes under attack.

So now, let's take a closer look at the physical makeup of the brain and at the disturbance in blood circulation that occurs during a stroke.

Brainstorming
About Your Brain

In some ways, your brain is a three-pound supercomputer. On the other hand, it is really not quite accurate to refer to the brain as a computer because it can do so much more than any man-made electronic device. To be sure, those of us who have worked with the computer stand in awe of its high-tech capacities. It is easy to become humbled by and respectful of the speed and accuracy of this electronic marvel.

Our brains, however, can perform many operations that the computer cannot. Though it may be slower, the human mind can duplicate computerlike functions, such as calculating and solving complex math problems and executing difficult verbal tasks. Also, electrical connections exist in the brain as they do in the computer. And there are complex chemical interactions involved in the brain's activities. Furthermore, the brain can control the body's functions, its actions and reactions; and it can think abstractly and creatively.

Comprising about 2 percent of your body weight, the brain does no mechanical work. But it *does* expend tremendous amounts of energy, as it transports complex chemical and electrical messages around in your head and to other parts of the body. As a consequence of this activity, the brain uses 15 percent of the output of blood of your heart; 20 percent of the available oxygen in your entire body; and much of your body's blood sugar, glucose! To put all this another way, the cerebral (brain) blood flow normally involves about three fourths of a quart of blood per minute—a great deal for only 2 percent of your body weight!

You might think of the blood as carrying the fuel that enables the brain to do all the necessary electrical and chemical work. The fuel is the oxygen and glucose. Without the fuel, the brain can't think, direct locomotion, monitor feelings, or operate the senses. Clearly, your brain needs plenty of blood to do its work! That's what the complex network of arteries and other blood vessels in your head is all about. Just as a real computer needs adequate amounts of electricity to run various programs, your brain requires sufficient circulation to enable you to think, react, and perform other tasks. The diagram below of the main arteries that deliver blood to various parts of your brain should give you some idea of how important brain circulation is.

But of course, this is only the tip of the brain's circulatory iceberg. In addition to these arteries, there are thousands of veins, capillaries, and other vessels that transport the essential blood fuels to every part of your body's God-given (and/or evolutionary) personal computer.

In addition to this comprehensive circuitry of vessels, the brain's circulatory system also has an exquisite mechanism to regulate the brain blood flow. Operating as a kind of self-regulatory protective device preventing surges of blood to or shortages of blood in the brain—much as electrical power strips do to prevent "spikes" of electricity from entering appliances or computers—this mechanism enables the amount of blood in the brain to remain remarkably constant. Whether you're resting or exercising, about the same volume of blood is always present in your head.

The reason for this self-regulating capacity of the brain boils down, in the end, to the body's capacity to protect itself. If the blood flow to the brain is interrupted for even five seconds, you can lose consciousness. A lack of blood to the brain for several minutes may cause permanent tissue damage—damage that deepens and spreads the longer that circulation is interrupted.

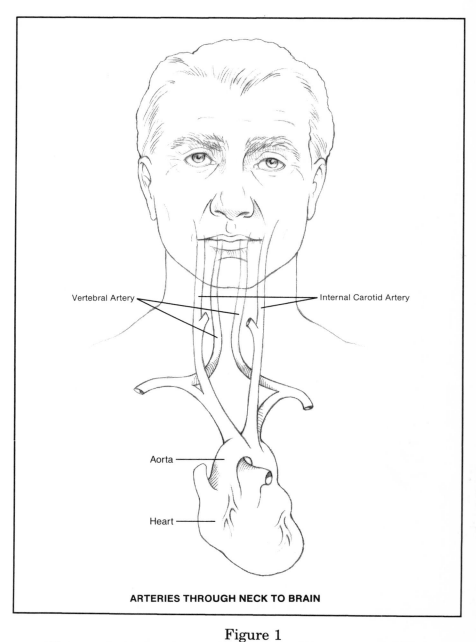

Vertebral Artery

Internal Carotid Artery

Aorta

Heart

ARTERIES THROUGH NECK TO BRAIN

Figure 1

Major Arteries in Your Head. *There are four principal arteries that bring blood to the brain. The two in the front of the neck are called the internal carotids (left and right). The two in the back of the neck are called the left and right vertebral arteries. In the brain, the vertebral arteries join and form the basilar artery. Within the brain, the basilar and the carotid arteries branch out and enter into connections with other vessels.*

On the other hand, recent sophisticated measuring methods have revealed that despite the consistency of the overall brain blood flow, there are regional differences, depending on what function the brain is performing at a given moment. For example, the visual centers of the brain receive more blood to perform their various tasks when you're awake than when you're asleep.

The brain also demonstrates tremendous strength and versatility in its ability to adapt to serious outside threats, including those that may eventually lead to death. One example is the occasional, remarkable recovery of people who have been trapped under icy water for long periods of time without access to air. The nutritional requirements of the brain are reduced in such an environment, so that for a time, a lessened blood flow to the brain is sufficient to supply its needs.

As an illustration, consider Tommy, aged twelve, who fell through the ice on a pond while playing hockey. He was submerged for about one hour before he was rescued. Resuscitation efforts were touch and go, but Tommy responded with a complete return to all normal functions. The medical explanation: His circulation delivered sufficient oxygen and glucose to meet at least the minimal requirements of his brain tissue.

Clearly, the brain has tremendous resources and protective capacities. But unfortunately, it has no inner defenses to protect itself against a stroke. Because a "brain attack" involves such a serious reduction of blood flow to the brain, the body's essential power source is shut down, and irreversible damage to the brain's electrical and chemical systems can occur.

What Happens
_____During a Stroke_____

As we saw in the first chapter, the various causes of stroke can be divided generally into four main categories that I want to deal with at this point: stationary clots that block off blood vessels (thrombosis); traveling clots that plug up vessels leading to the brain (embolisms); bleeding vessels in the brain (intracerebral hemorrhaging); and bleeding in the spaces between the layers of tissues that house the brain (subarachnoid hemorrhaging).

What types of stroke tend to be the most frequent? Blockages of the blood vessels account for about two thirds of all stroke deaths. Bleeding into the brain (intracerebral hemorrhaging), the second major cause of death, results in about 15 percent of the fatalities. Even though hemorrhaging strokes hit less frequently than blockage strokes, they are more dangerous because they do their damage in two ways: They shut off blood to the brain *and* they flood surrounding brain tissue with escaping blood.

Even for experienced medical specialists, it may be impossible to tell whether blockage or hemorrhaging is involved when stroke first occurs. A CAT scan or MRI (magnetic resonance imaging) is required for that determination. It's enough for you to remember that *all* types of stroke are potentially deadly and *all* can produce serious disabilities if swift countermeasures aren't taken.

Now, to give you an idea about exactly what happens in the victim's head when stroke strikes, here are four representative scenarios, two involving a blockage and two a hemorrhage.

Attack 1: Sam's surreptitious stationary clot. Sam, who was sixty-two years old, had been heading for a stroke for a long time. Outwardly, he appeared in good health. But when he first had his cholesterol and other blood lipids tested when he was in his late forties, a problem became evident.

The lab tests revealed that his total cholesterol was 290 mg/dl (milligrams per deciliter), well above the 200-mg/dl ceiling recommended today. Also, his "good" cholesterol—the high-density lipoprotein (HDL) measurement, which is associated with lower cardiovascular risk—was relatively low, about 40 mg/dl. In general, the higher the HDL, the greater the protection against heart attacks and strokes. It is desirable for the HDLs in a man over sixty to be above 45.

These findings suggested that Sam was in danger. His high-fat diet and high cholesterol levels had accelerated the steady process of atherosclerosis—the narrowing of his arterial blood vessels with fatty deposits. (As with most people, the process in Sam had begun in childhood.) As a result of the findings,

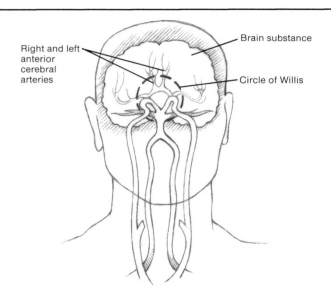

ILLUSTRATION OF STROKE DUE TO AN OBSTRUCTION OF ANTERIOR CEREBRAL ARTERY

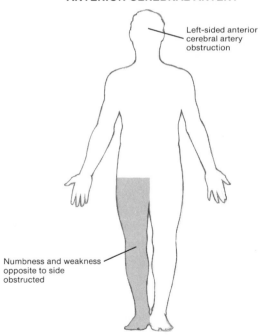

LEFT-SIDED OBSTRUCTION CAUSES RIGHT LOWER EXTREMITY DISABILITY

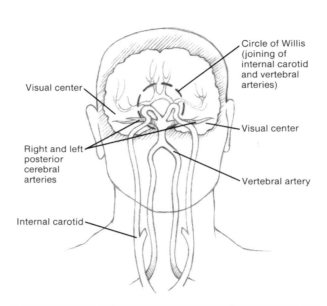

Visual center

Circle of Willis
(joining of
internal carotid
and vertebral
arteries)

Visual center

Right and left
posterior
cerebral
arteries

Vertebral artery

Internal carotid

ILLUSTRATION OF STROKE DUE TO OBSTRUCTION OF POSTERIOR CEREBRAL ARTERY

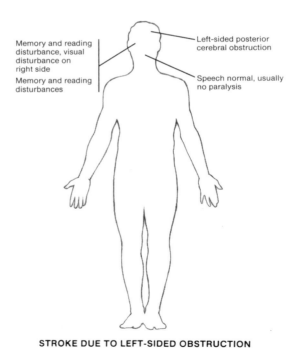

Memory and reading
disturbance, visual
disturbance on
right side

Memory and reading
disturbances

Left-sided posterior
cerebral obstruction

Speech normal, usually
no paralysis

STROKE DUE TO LEFT-SIDED OBSTRUCTION

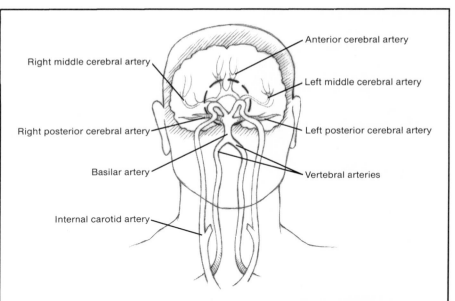

Right middle cerebral artery

Anterior cerebral artery

Left middle cerebral artery

Right posterior cerebral artery

Left posterior cerebral artery

Basilar artery

Vertebral arteries

Internal carotid artery

ILLUSTRATION OF STROKE DUE TO OBSTRUCTION OF MIDDLE CEREBRAL ARTERY

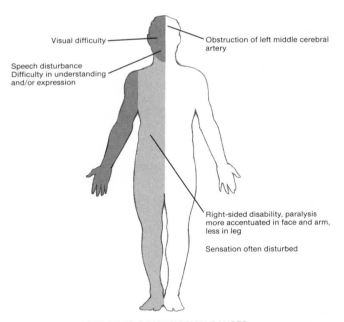

Visual difficulty

Obstruction of left middle cerebral artery

Speech disturbance
Difficulty in understanding
and/or expression

Right-sided disability, paralysis
more accentuated in face and arm,
less in leg

Sensation often disturbed

LEFT-SIDED OBSTRUCTION CAUSES RIGHT-SIDED DISABILITY

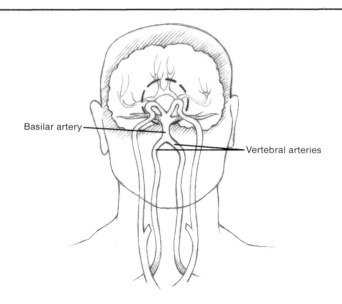

Basilar artery

Vertebral arteries

ILLUSTRATION OF STROKE DUE TO OBSTRUCTION OF VERTEBROBASILAR ARTERY

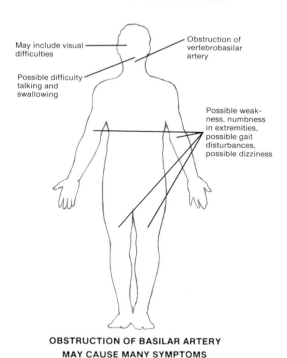

May include visual difficulties

Obstruction of vertebrobasilar artery

Possible difficulty talking and swallowing

Possible weakness, numbness in extremities, possible gait disturbances, possible dizziness

**OBSTRUCTION OF BASILAR ARTERY
MAY CAUSE MANY SYMPTOMS**

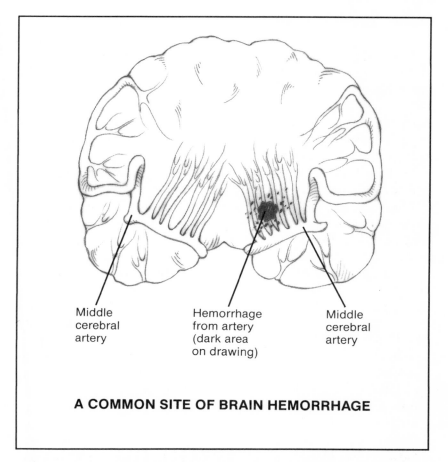

Middle
cerebral
artery

Hemorrhage
from artery
(dark area
on drawing)

Middle
cerebral
artery

A COMMON SITE OF BRAIN HEMORRHAGE

Sam's physician identified him as a candidate for cardiovascular trouble. The prescription: a strict low-cholesterol diet initially and later, if necessary, cholesterol-lowering medications.

But Sam didn't take his doctor's advice very seriously. He neglected the recommended diet in favor of his normal high-fat fare and also failed to take his medications regularly. "I feel fine, so why worry?" was his philosophy.

If you had talked to Sam a few seconds before the cutoff of blood to his brain, he would have told you, "I *still* feel fine!" He was diligently finishing up some paperwork in his office at the end of the day, and though he was tired, he didn't sense that anything unusual was about to happen.

Obviously, though, Sam *wasn't* fine, and something unusual *was* about to happen. He was on the verge of a stroke that was capable of causing serious physical and mental impairment, and perhaps even death. The blood flow to the left side of his brain became impaired, and he lost his ability to speak. The muscles of the right side of his face became weak and he partially lost the use of his right arm. As those who have experienced a stroke know, signals like these are much more arresting and terrifying than any alarm bells.

Luckily, Sam had learned enough from his physician to recognize that something serious and dangerous was happening to him. Based on what he had read and heard, he immediately suspected a stroke and, using a pencil and pad of paper to communicate, he urged a fellow worker to get him to a hospital as quickly as possible.

The speed with which he was rushed to the emergency room helped to head off the worst effects of the stroke. Now, a year later, Sam has fully recovered his ability to speak and use his right arm, and most of the paralysis on the right side of his face has disappeared.

What lessons can we learn from Sam's experience? On the positive side, he acted quickly when the stroke hit. As a result, as with Dr. Robert M., described in the previous chapter, the damage done by the attack was minimized.

But Sam might have avoided it altogether if he had just followed his physician's advice about diet and medication. Studies have shown that a low-fat diet, which may be combined with medications to lower blood fats, can stop the progress of atherosclerosis and may even *reverse* it!

In other words, by following his physician's instructions, Sam might have succeeded in reducing the fatty plaque buildup that was narrowing his carotid artery and setting him up for the clot, or thrombus, that eventually triggered the stroke. The same can be said for others—perhaps including you—who may not yet have suffered a stroke, but who may be at risk for a blockage type of brain attack.

Attack 2: how Helen might have avoided a tragic brain hemorrhage. Helen, who was in her mid-forties, wasn't as lucky as Sam. For more than twenty years, she had experienced high blood pressure (hypertension). Her blood pressure measurements during that period averaged about 165/105 mm Hg (millimeters of mercury). (Normal adult blood pressure is under 140/90. More on blood pressure in Chapter Five.)

Helen had been to see a doctor a few times and had been diagnosed as a "hypertensive," or one who has high blood pressure disease. But she had rarely taken the prescribed medications that would have brought her readings down to normal.

"Those pills make me feel like I'm going to the bathroom all the time," she complained, referring to her antihypertensive diuretic medication. Her prescribed medication, indeed, encouraged urination to lower the volume of fluid and salt in the body and thus lower blood pressure.

Although her doctor suggested other medications, his description of possible side effects discouraged Helen, and so she elected just to live with her high blood pressure. "After all, I don't *feel* bad with it, so I guess I'll get along all right," she rationalized. "Besides, I don't have headaches." She didn't realize that headaches are a very late symptom in hypertension. *Indeed, most patients with high blood pressure never have headaches.*

She never accepted the warning from her physician that hypertension is by nature a silent, symptomless disease, which gradually ravages the body's blood vessels over years or decades. The final result of uncontrolled hypertension is often a stroke—in some cases a hemorrhagic or bleeding stroke—and that's exactly what happened to Helen.

Although she was unaware of what was happening inside her body, the steady, excessively high pressure in her arteries began to damage the walls of the arteries in the brain. In some parts of her body, the roughening of the walls encouraged the development of atherosclerosis, or clogging of the arteries. But even before the danger with atherosclerosis became apparent, another, more ominous result of her hypertension took its toll.

Inside Helen's brain, small defects in her arteries began to occur due to the high blood pressure. The walls of some areas of these arteries became thin and balloonlike. The balloonlike dilation of the weakened arteries was unable to withstand the incessant high blood pressure. Finally, the walls in one section of her brain artery burst and a "spontaneous intracerebral hemorrhage" resulted. In plain English, this means that the blood escaped from the vessels and spread out in the surrounding brain tissue, severely damaging it. Also, the blood flow to part of the right side of her brain was interrupted by this leakage.

As with many who suffer a blockage-type stroke, the interruption of blood flow resulting from Helen's hemorrhage caused paralysis in her arm and face and lower extremity.

Helen also experienced other reactions, including headache, nausea, and an increasing stiffness in her neck. On the way to the hospital, she lost consciousness—another sign that a vessel in her brain was hemorrhaging.

Helen began to undergo treatment, including medication to lower her blood pressure, within about two hours of the time that her stroke struck, and that was *very* fortunate for her. Without treatment, about 40 percent of those who have a bleeding stroke die, as compared with a much lower 10–15 percent of those who die from an untreated blockage-type stroke. The reason for the tremendous danger with a brain hemorrhage attack is that the escaping blood damages brain tissue at the same time that normal blood flow is being interrupted.

Helen is still recovering from her stroke, and will probably remain somewhat impaired. She lived only because she made it to the hospital fairly quickly and received intensive care. The tragedy is that if she had only taken her physician's advice and begun to control her high blood pressure years earlier, she would probably never have suffered a stroke at all.

Attack 3: the traveling plug. John, who was fifty-five years of age, was a successful farmer who believed in the virtues of a "good old-fashioned American diet." He had eaten bacon and eggs and buttered toast for breakfast every day of his life until he was fifty years of age. At that time, he suffered his first heart attack. After his second heart attack two years later, he realized that the good old American diet he had been consuming was not so good after all.

One signal that things were not in perfect working order was an abnormal rhythm in his heartbeat, a condition called auricular fibrillation. Then one morning he failed to get out of bed at his usual early hour. His wife discovered that he had suffered a stroke that had paralyzed his right side and impaired his speech.

Specifically, John had suffered a stroke from a traveling plug, or embolism. A clot had developed within his damaged, irregularly beating heart. Then it had broken off the heart wall and floated through his vessels until finally, the clot stopped up an artery in the brain.

Could this tragedy have been prevented? Yes indeed! Medication to control the rhythm of the heart is widely available, and a simple dose of one aspirin a day might have averted the stroke. The aspirin might have prevented the formation of the clot.

Attack 4: bleeding in the space between the two tissue layers covering the brain.

Peter, an eighteen-year-old athlete, became unconscious while playing football. He was taken to the hospital where various examinations, including a CAT scan, revealed he had suffered a rupture of a weak artery at the base of his brain. The weakness involved the thin, balloon-like bulge in the artery called an aneurysm.

The physicians on duty performed emergency surgery to tie off the aneurysm and prevent further loss of blood. Then, special medications and weeks of hospitalization were necessary. Yet despite the serious nature of the attack, Peter has recovered fully.

This young man's case illustrates the bleeding attack in the brain that we call a subarachnoid hemorrhage. The main lesson: Speed in beginning emergency surgery was essential in warding off further injury and saving Peter's life.

Although these examples of stroke are different in many ways, there are also a number of important similarities. First of all, it is necessary to act quickly when the symptoms of stroke become apparent. Just as important, it's essential for those of you who have not suffered from a stroke to realize that you can act *now* to head one off. In the following chapter, we will explore some of the "rules of risk" that will help you reduce the chances that this ominous threat will strike you.

Chapter Three

The Rules of Risk

Living is a risky business. Through our lives, our health is subject to the laws of chance and probability. Our genetic makeup and environmental influences determine who will get what disease and when it will come. In the future, it will be possible to alter our genetics, but our best chance presently for the good life is to limit risks imposed by our environment.

Much of any successful life is devoted to the management of risk. Achievement in one's career is linked closely to minimizing the chances that a client will be displeased or a job lost. A long, happy marriage depends on reducing those influences that promote incompatibility and conflict. Those thrust into war learn to keep their heads down and to watch paths carefully for booby traps.

It is the same with one's health. A long, disease-free life depends heavily on eliminating or limiting various *risk factors*—or those events and influences that increase the probability that a certain illness will occur. The purpose of this chapter is to introduce you to the major risk factors that increase the likelihood of stroke—and to help you start minimizing those risks that could eventually jeopardize your health and life.

A person who has already suffered a stroke has the biological makeup predisposing him or her to another stroke unless that makeup is altered. Consequently, this discussion is directed both at those who have never had a stroke, and *also* at those who have suffered stroke and need to prevent a recurrence.

Some of these "rules of risk" for stroke will be dealt with more extensively in later chapters. For now, we will focus on acquiring an overview of the main risk factors and on how you can evaluate your own personal risk for stroke.

What Are the Risk Factors for Stroke?

By identifying the risk factors in your life—and doing something about them—you can greatly reduce the odds that you'll suffer a stroke. But first, it is important to understand some general principles.

The presence of one risk factor or several doesn't necessarily mean that a stroke will occur. By the same token, the absence of any of the following risk factors does not mean a person won't suffer a stroke. But the *probability* of a stroke's occurring definitely does increase with the presence of one or more of the risk factors.

Also, an important principle relating to risk factors is that one and one can make three. In other words, if two risk factors are present, the *cumulative* effect is greater than the total impact of each considered independently. For example, a person who has high blood pressure *and* high cholesterol is more than twice as likely to have a stroke as a person who has only one of those conditions.

You will also see that some of these risk factors can be influenced or changed more easily than others. For example, you obviously can't change your sex, medical history of stroke, family history, or age. On the other hand, you *can* take steps to eliminate or reduce high blood pressure (hypertension), cigarette smoking, and fatty foods.

To help you focus on those factors you can alter, I have

divided the risk factors into the two separate categories: first, those you can change; then, those you can't change—but may be able to modify.

Finally, I suggest that you use these brief descriptions of the main risk factors for stroke as a kind of checklist to see where you stand. Then, after we have gone over each of them, you'll learn more about how to evaluate yourself.

Risk Factors You Can Change

Risk factor 1: high blood pressure. High blood pressure, medically referred to as hypertension, is a very important risk factor for all types of stroke, especially those caused by artery blockage and hemorrhaging into the brain.

Blood pressure is typically measured by wrapping a special device called a sphygmomanometer around the upper arm, pumping it up, and getting a reading in millimeters of mercury, or mm Hg. The result is expressed in two numbers, separated by a slash, such as 120/80 (normal blood pressure).

The first (or upper) number is called the "systolic" pressure; it reflects the pressure of blood against the walls of an artery as the heart pumps. The second (or lower) figure is the "diastolic" pressure, which indicates the pressure of the blood against the arterial walls while the heart is resting (between beats). This figure represents the elasticity of the arteries.

The classic Framingham study is the source of much of our knowledge regarding risk factors. Framingham is a town in Massachusetts where thousands of "average" people have been examined periodically since 1948. The people of Framingham who have suffered heart attacks, strokes, and many other illnesses have been studied in relation to their alcohol consumption, high blood pressure, smoking, and other external environmental factors.

At Framingham and other sites around the world where studies have been conducted, there is strong evidence that a high systolic reading or a high diastolic reading, *and* a combination of both readings are very significant risk factors for stroke. In other words, if you have a blood pressure above 140/90 mm Hg, your chances of having a stroke are higher—and the risk increases as the blood pressure increases. Conversely, if you have normal blood pressure, the odds are much less that you'll have a stroke.

The issue of high blood pressure disease—and how to control it—is so important that I'll be dealing with it in much more detail in Chapter Five.

Risk factor 2: smoking. There is overwhelming scientific evidence that cigarette smoking is a major risk factor for strokes that are caused by blockage of an artery to the brain.

Some smokers would like to follow the lead of Jean Nicot, a French diplomat who introduced tobacco into France and from whose name the word "nicotine" derives. He thought smoking had beneficial medicinal value. Although he was quite wrong, his arguments helped create a health scourge that has claimed millions of lives by lung cancer, heart attacks, strokes, emphysema, and other diseases. The habit is so addictive that even heavy increases in cigarette taxes, beginning with the first levy back in 1614, have failed to curb the use of tobacco. Taxes, disease, and death remain the scourge of the smoker!

The bad news linking cigarettes and stroke is particularly disturbing: Smoking increases the risk of stroke at least 2 to 3 times, with the risk rising 1.5 times for every ten cigarettes smoked. The good news is that the effects of smoking are reversible. Stop smoking, and the risk will begin to disappear. Specifically, according to the Framingham investigation, refraining from cigarettes almost immediately reduces the risk significantly. After five nonsmoking years, the risk of the former smokers was the same as that for nonsmokers.

A further word of warning: Today, young females are the most likely new smokers and are twice as likely as teenage boys to smoke daily. In particular, women who smoke *and* use the birth control pill are at significantly higher risk for stroke than other people.

Under the supervision of the National Cancer Institute and the American Cancer Society, a seven-year project known as the Stop Smoking Intervention Study has been launched in seventeen states. The goal is to save 1.2 million Americans from smoking-related deaths and to prevent 2 million young people from starting to smoke.

Risk factor 3: diabetes mellitus. Diabetes is a risk factor for all types of stroke. Although there is the hope that ongoing research will significantly reduce the risk of stroke associated with diabetes, currently the dangers of this disease continue at a high level.

Diabetes ages the arteries of the body prematurely and thereby increases the risk of stroke. Many physicians who specialize in diabetes advocate better control of the blood sugar and low-fat diets as a way to reduce all the complications of diabetes, including the premature aging of the arteries.

Risk factor 4: cholesterol. Our government and the medical profession have jointly declared war on cholesterol. Why? Overwhelming scientific data have been accumulated in studies showing that increased levels of cholesterol contribute to the buildup of fatty plaques in the arteries. This process is known as atherosclerosis, or, in popular parlance, "hardening of the arteries." There is also strong anthropological evidence from S. Boyd Eaton and his co-workers at Emory University in Atlanta that low serum cholesterol levels parallel the paucity of atherosclerosis in many societies. Hardening of the arteries is the major cause of heart attacks and strokes.

Is everyone at risk for excessive cholesterol in the blood? The answer is no. Some of us can handle cholesterol, but most can't. Part of the answer as to who can or can't handle cholesterol resides in the HDL and LDL story, which will be explored in Chapter Six.

Risk factor 5: alcoholism and other substance abuse. Drinking alcohol, at least in modest amounts, has at times been recommended to the public as a practice capable of reducing the risk of heart disease. But new studies reveal there may be an undesirable downside to alcohol consumption, and particularly to heavy alcohol consumption.

Binge drinking has been associated with irregular heart action, heart muscle damage, and high blood pressure. Even three drinks a day has been found to increase the risk of high blood pressure. Men who are heavy drinkers (more than three or four drinks daily) have more than four times the risk for stroke as nondrinkers.

Exactly how much is safe to drink? It has been suggested by hypertension expert Dr. Norman Kaplan that the threshold for "safe" consumption of alcohol is no more than about one ounce of pure alcohol per day. This translates, according to Kaplan, into about two beers, two glasses of wine, or two mixed drinks per day. Any amount above that may significantly increase the risk of high blood pressure and stroke.

Caution: Even minimal amounts of alcohol impair the judgment and reaction time of operators of all kinds of vehicles, from bicycles, to automobiles, to airplanes. There is a risk from alcohol not only for the user and abuser, but for the innocent public as well. Impaired reaction time caused by drinking can lead to accidental injury and death of innocents.

Other types of substance abuse, especially involving cocaine, also increases the risk of stroke. Cocaine-related stroke is the most common kind occurring in young adults. Cocaine elevates the blood pressure and can induce hemorrhaging in the brain. All three of the major ways in which the drug is used have been implicated:

* Smoking "crack," or the purified form of cocaine

* "Snorting" through the nose

* Injecting the drug into the veins or muscles

In one study of forty-seven cases of stroke in young abusers, the majority suffered hemorrhage in the brain because of blood pressure elevation.

Risk factor 6: obesity. Obesity, or excess body fat that causes puffiness, pudginess, and potbellies, is a major enemy of health. More specifically, obesity can be considered a risk factor for stroke because it is related to hypertension, and hence to hemorrhaging in the brain.

Obesity is the most prevalent nutritional disorder in prosperous communities. It is the result of an energy imbalance leading to the storage of energy as fat. In most instances, one can tell at a glance who is obese. This is called the mirror test. There are two patterns of obesity that are common. The "beer belly" or apple shape is one in which excess fat is in the abdominal area. The other is the pear-shape type of obesity where deposits of fat are around the hips and buttocks. Height and weight tables, measuring skinfold with caliper, and underwater weighing are other techniques used to define who is and who is not obese. Height-weight tables give a rough estimate of normal values.

Recent studies have revealed that upper body fat—on the abdomen and higher on the trunk—is associated with cardiovascular problems more than is lower body fat, on the legs or hips. Of course, the accumulation of fat in certain sites on the body is more dependent on your genetic background than anything else.

Slimming down is big business that is not necessarily good business. The basic way to lose weight is to reduce the amount of food eaten on a consistent basis. Unfortunately, the MIS triad—*mis*information, *mis*leading claims, and *mis*understandings—contributes to a fourth MIS—the *mis*ery of the obese person.

If your intake of food exceeds the amount used as fuel for your body activities, weight gain and obesity will result. The laws of thermodynamics can't be repealed. An eating and exercise plan without crash diets and gimmicks will work.

So if you are at all obese—and especially if you tend to put your weight on around the middle or the chest—you should lose those extra pounds as soon as possible. When they are gone, your risk for stroke, as well as other health problems, will be lower. The maintenance of a lower weight requires resolve, dedication, and, above all, discipline. Control of weight usually has beneficial effects on high blood pressure, diabetes and blood fats.

Risk factor 7: sedentary life-style. Another enemy of fitness and potent risk factor for stroke is a sedentary life-style. Minimal physical activity can contribute to obstructions in some of our important arteries. But increasing the level of exercise—along with a low-fat diet, cessation of smoking, and better stress management—has actually been shown to *reverse* the process of atherosclerosis. (More on this later.)

It is doubtful that exercise alone can achieve this result: Witness the untimely death of the running guru Jim Fixx from a heart attack. Exercise doesn't "burn off" the cholesterol deposits in your arteries. Still, exercise helps in weight control, contributes to a feeling of well-being due to the increased circulation of endorphins (morphinelike substances produced by the brain), and serves as an outlet for tension.

Risk Factors That Are Hard or Impossible to Change

Although you can't eliminate the following risk factors by life-style changes as you can the previous seven, you *can* mitigate or influence their impact. The main way to reduce the danger posed by these factors is to eliminate or lessen other risk factors that are in your power to control. Remember: With risk factors, one plus one is more than two. The more factors you have, the greater the negative effect is multiplied or magnified. Conversely, the fewer you have, the better are your chances of avoiding stroke.

Risk factor 8: noises in the neck. Your physician may be able to detect a murmur or other regular sound (a "bruit"; pronounced brū-ē') when he places a stethoscope over one of the large carotid arteries on each side of the neck. The sound is caused as blood rushes through the artery, which has been narrowed as a result of atherosclerosis. (The sound, by the way, resembles that produced by blowing on the top of a soda bottle.) Studies have revealed that 3–5 percent of those over forty-five years of age have such a bruit, and the incidence of these sounds increases with age.

The key message for our purposes is that the presence of these bruits, including those without any accompanying symptoms, is an important risk factor for stroke. The annual stroke rate among those who have asymptomatic bruits, and who are not being treated to prevent stroke or heart disease, is higher than for those who don't have bruits. Furthermore, there is a higher risk among those with such bruits who are known to have at least 70-percent blockage of a neck artery going to the brain.

When detected, bruits are usually investigated by ultrasound studies called Dopplers and by arteriograms—X rays of the arteries of the neck.

Risk factor 9: irregular beat of the heart. The normal heart beats regularly at a rate of about 60 to 100 beats per minute. One of the most common irregularities of the heart-beat, which has been associated with an increased incidence of stroke, is called auricular fibrillation. This irregularity may be associated with rheumatic fever, overactivity of the thyroid gland, and advancing age. This type of irregularity leads to the formation of clots within the heart chamber, which can break off and plug an artery to the brain. The end result is a stroke due to a traveling plug—an embolus.

The diagnosis of auricular fibrillation (or atrial fibrillation, as it is also known) is associated with a great risk for stroke. In recent years, however, the use of medication as simple as aspirin has been shown to prevent clot formation and hence embolization. Established by an electrocardiogram, more than one million Americans have auricular fibrillation.

In more complex situations, more powerful medications (the anticoagulants, or clot preventers) are used. One of them, Cou-madin, works by blocking the action of vitamin K so that blood cannot clot as readily. It is clear that anticoagulant therapy is effective in reducing the risk of stroke in patients with auricular fibrillation.

Risk factor 10: the ministroke signal. One of the clear signs that a full-fledged stroke may be on the horizon is a kind of "ministroke," or what physicians call a "transient ischemic attack" (TIA for short). A TIA involves the temporary interruption of blood flow to the brain, often with strokelike symptoms, such as speech problems or weakness. After a short time, however, bodily functions return to normal.

It is wise not to become complacent after recovery from a ministroke. Action is required. Approximately 10 percent of all patients with stroke have had a preceding ministroke.

We will deal with this important subject in more detail in the following chapter—and among other things, help you dis-tinguish a TIA from common dizziness and fainting.

Risk factor 11: advancing age. Aging is a definite risk factor for stroke. One of the reasons that stroke incidence increases with age is the damage suffered by the arteries as we get older. The arteries become more rigid, or less pliable and elastic, with aging. Consequently, they become more susceptible to obstructions and hemorrhaging. Atherosclerosis in human beings is a tissue response that evolves over decades. Many factors contribute, such as genetics, diet, inflammations, and hormonal changes.

Extensive research is continuing into the impact of aging on stroke. In the meantime, the best way to reduce that impact is to reduce the effect of those risk factors that you can control—and that become more dangerous as you grow older.

Risk factor 12: the catch-all category. There are a number of other risk factors that are often associated with an increased incidence of stroke, even though these points may not be listed among the most pressing issues confronting us.

Some of the most important factors in our final, catch-all category are:

* *Male gender.* More men than women tend to have strokes, at least up to about age seventy-five. After that, the occurrence of the disease begins to level off between the sexes. Then, strokes in females are more frequent. Approximately 90,000 women of all ages die of stroke each year.

* *"Rich blood."* Polycythemia, or "rich blood," is a condition in which the number of red blood cells is higher than normal, and the blood becomes very thick or viscous. This situation is associated with strokes resulting from a blockage of blood flow in the brain arteries, since the blood is more coaguable.

  High hemoglobin values in the blood—an indicator of polycythemia—can double the risk of stroke when the measurements are considerably more than 15 grams per deciliter (g/dl) in men and more than 14 g/dl in women. Medications can reduce this risk factor.

* *Antibody reactions.* The body manufactures substances called antibodies that react to foreign chemicals. Rarely,

the body makes antibodies to our own tissues causing what we call auto-immune diseases. These diseases attack arteries and are an unusual cause of stroke.

⋆ *Race.* Blacks over age thirty-five suffer strokes about twice as often as whites. Why is that? Among other things, blacks have more diabetes and hypertension than whites; those two conditions, as we have seen, are associated with increased risk of stroke.

But even when diabetes and high blood pressure are factored out, blacks still have a significantly higher incidence of stroke than whites. For example, according to the National Health and Nutrition Examination Survey of 1971–75, black women had 1.4 times the estimated stroke risk of white women—*without* considering hypertension or diabetes. The death rate for black women due to stroke is 80 percent higher than for white women.

⋆ *Family or genetic factors.* A family history of stroke may influence a person's chances of having a stroke, though clear conclusions are generally not available yet on this subject. It may be that a tendency toward hypertension is the most important familial factor.

⋆ *A prior stroke.* Having one stroke predisposes a person toward having another. According to the Framingham study, for instance, more than one fifth of the men and women who had one stroke had a second one.

⋆ *Gout.* This condition, which can be overcome through medications, is caused by the accumulation of a protein end product, known as uric acid, in the blood. The elevation of uric acid can cause painful joint disease.

Once detected, however, gout can be cured by the use of certain drugs. So gout, in effect, is a disease of choice. If you could choose a disease, this would be the one to have, because it's virtually completely reversible!

These, then, are the major risk factors that have been associated with an increased chance of having a stroke. Other controllable, though relatively rare, problems in North America and Europe include infections that lead to stroke. Infections such as tuberculosis, malaria, and syphilis have been associated with increased incidence of stroke.

Now that you are aware of the major risk factors, how can you *use* them in reducing your own chances of being attacked by this dread disease? The answer lies in the application of the "rules of risk."

Applying the
Rules of Risk

The Stroke Risk Factor Prediction Chart is used to estimate the possibility or likelihood of stroke over a ten-year period in those aged fifty-four to eighty-six. The chart was prepared by researchers from the Framingham study. Our nation has had many public health successes. The Framingham study is destined to be one of the greatest. The chart is based on data obtained from 2,372 men and 3,362 women. Eight risk factors were used. They include some but not all risk factors:

* Age and sex

* Systolic blood pressure—the upper figure of your blood pressure (see Chapter Five)

* Use of medicine for blood pressure control

* Diabetes diagnosis

* Cigarette smoking

* History of irregular heart action

* Enlarged left ventricle of the heart as determined by the electrocardiograph

* Cardiovascular disease (CVD)—history of a heart attack or chest pains due to poor circulation to the heart (angina)

Your physician can give you explanations about those factors that you are not likely to be aware of, such as enlargement of the left ventricle of the heart. Using the Stroke Risk Factor Prevention Chart, add up the points that apply to you and

Table 1. Stroke Risk Factor Prediction Chart

1. FIND POINTS FOR EACH RISK FACTOR

Men

Age	SBP	Hyp Rx	Diabetes
54–56 = 0	95–105 = 0	No = 0	No = 0
57–59 = 1	106–116 = 1	Yes = 2	Yes = 2
60–62 = 2	117–126 = 2		
63–65 = 3	127–137 = 3	**Cigs**	**CVD**
66–68 = 4	138–148 = 4	No = 0	No = 0
69–71 = 5	149–159 = 5	Yes = 3	Yes = 3
72–74 = 6	160–170 = 6		
75–77 = 7	171–181 = 7	**AF**	**LVH**
78–80 = 8	182–191 = 8	No = 0	No = 0
81–83 = 9	192–202 = 9	Yes = 4	Yes = 6
84–86 = 10	203–213 = 10		

Women

Age	SBP	Hyp Rx	Diabetes
54–56 = 0	95–104 = 0	No = 0	No = 0
57–59 = 1	105–114 = 1	If yes, see below	Yes = 3
60–62 = 2	115–124 = 2		
63–65 = 3	125–134 = 3	**Cigs**	**CVD**
66–68 = 4	135–144 = 4	No = 0	No = 0
69–71 = 5	145–154 = 5	Yes = 3	Yes = 2
72–74 = 6	155–164 = 6		
75–77 = 7	165–174 = 7	**AF**	**LVH**
78–80 = 8	175–184 = 8	No = 0	No = 0
81–83 = 9	185–194 = 9	Yes = 6	Yes = 4
84–86 = 10	195–204 = 10		

Women: If currently under antihypertensive therapy add the following points depending on SBP level.

SPB	95–104	105–114	115–124	125–134	135–144	145–154	155–164	165–174	175–184	185–194	195–204
Points	6	5	5	4	3	3	2	1	1	0	0

2. SUM POINTS FOR ALL RISK FACTORS

____ + ____ + ____ + ____ + ____ + ____ + ____ + ____ = ____
Age   SBP   Hp Rx   Diabetes Cigs   CVD   AF   LVH   Point total

3. LOOK UP RISK CORRESPONDING TO POINT TOTAL

Men 10-yr.

Pts.	Prob.	Pts.	Prob.	Pts.	Prob.
1	2.6%	11	11.2%	21	41.7%
2	3.0%	12	12.9%	22	46.6%
3	3.5%	13	14.8%	23	51.8%
4	4.0%	14	17.0%	24	57.3%
5	4.7%	15	19.5%	25	62.8%
6	5.4%	16	22.4%	26	68.4%
7	6.3%	17	25.5%	27	73.8%
8	7.3%	18	29.0%	28	79.0%
9	8.4%	19	32.9%	29	83.7%
10	9.7%	20	37.1%	30	87.9%

Women 10-yr.

Pts.	Prob.	Pts.	Prob.	Pts.	Prob.
1	1.1%	11	7.6%	21	43.4%
2	1.3%	12	9.2%	22	50.0%
3	1.6%	13	11.1%	23	57.0%
4	2.0%	14	13.3%	24	64.2%
5	2.4%	15	16.0%	25	71.4%
6	2.9%	16	19.1%	26	78.2%
7	3.5%	17	22.8%	27	84.4%
8	4.3%	18	27.0%		
9	5.2%	19	31.9%		
10	6.3%	20	37.3%		

4. COMPARE TO AVERAGE 10-YEAR RISK

Avg. 10-yr. prob. by age

Men		Women	
55–59	5.9%	55–59	3.0%
60–64	7.8%	60–64	4.7%
65–69	11.0%	65–69	7.2%
70–74	13.7%	70–74	10.9%
75–79	18.0%	75–79	15.5%
80–84	22.3%	80–84	23.9%

Key for symbols

SBP Systolic blood pressure—the upper figure of your BP.
Hyp Rx Under antihypertensive therapy?
Diabetes History of diabetes?
Cigs Smokes cigarettes?
CVD History of myocardial infarction, angina pectoris, coronary insufficiency, intermittent claudication, or congestive heart failure?
AF History of atrial fibrillation?
LVH Left ventricular hypertrophy on ECG?

NOTE: This chart was prepared with the help of William B. Kannel, M.D., Professor of Medicine and Public Health, and Ralph D'Agostino, Ph.D., Head, Department of Mathematics, both at Boston University; Kaaven Anderson, Ph.D., Statistician, NHLBI, Framingham study; Daniel McGee, Ph.D., Associate Professor, University of Arizona. Reproduced with permission. Risk Factor Prediction Kit, 1990, © American Heart Association.

NOTE: Reprinted, by permission, from *Patient Care*, October 30, 1991, p. 16.

determine your risk corresponding to the point total. The purpose of the chart is to motivate a person to modify risk factors and to reduce the risk.

Example 1: Mr. G.F. is sixty-seven. His blood pressure is 130/80. He does not have treatment for high blood pressure or diabetes. There is no history of CVD (heart disease), no AF (irregular heart action), and no LVH (enlarged heart). His score is 4 points for age plus 3 points for SBP (systolic blood pressure). He has no points for treatment of hypertension (Hyp Rx), diabetes, smoking, heart disease (CVD), irregular heart action (AF), or enlarged heart (LVH). His total points are therefore 7. He has a very low risk of having a stroke—6.3 percent in his next ten years of life. Compared with an average ten-year risk at his age of 11 percent, G.F. is doing quite well and faces no extraordinary risks.

Example 2: Mrs. D.B. is fifty-eight and being treated for high blood pressure. Her electrocardiogram reveals evidence of an enlarged heart. Her blood pressure (BP) is 150/80. Her age gives her 1 point; her systolic BP gives her 5 points; she gets 3 points for high blood pressure treatment. She gets 3 points for smoking; she gets no points for diabetes, heart disease, or irregular heart action, but does get 4 points for an enlarged heart. Her total points are 15. According to the chart she stands a 16-percent risk of stroke within ten years. If she stopped smoking and reduced her blood pressure somewhat, she could lower her total points to 9. That would lower her stroke risk to 5.2 percent within ten years, which represents about a two-thirds reduction of risk!

Note: The above rules of risk apply to *everyone.* This includes (1) those who haven't had a stroke, but feel they may be predisposed to this disease, *and* (2) those who have already had one stroke and want to prevent a second.

As indicated in the above-listed categories, it is important at the outset to distinguish those risk factors you *can* control from those you *can't.* For example, you obviously can't change your age, family history, or personal experience of a prior stroke. On the other hand, you *can* minimize the impact of these fixed risk factors by reducing the influence of factors that can be altered. So, controlling hypertension, stopping cigarette smoking, or countering hardening of the arteries will lessen the risk you run because of your age or family history.

The presence of *any* of the above risk factors should serve as a warning and stimulus to action. If possible, steps should be taken to limit or eliminate *all* those factors that can be influenced. The reason for such comprehensive, close attention to the risk issue is that any one of these factors, with or without the others, can trigger a stroke.

Even with such an all-encompassing personal strategy, however, you should think in terms of certain *priorities* of action, because certain risk factors do raise the odds against you more than others. To this end, one should order a personal prevention plan according to what might be called the top five threats: TIAs, high blood pressure, hardening of the arteries, smoking, and too much alcohol.

The next three chapters of this book have been organized to follow an all-important, three-pronged attack. As you read, you'll move naturally through the three steps that will enable you to apply the rules of risk most effectively in order to achieve *risk reversal.*

Step 1: Under your physician's supervision, respond immediately to any ministroke (TIA) signal.

Step 2: Lower high blood pressure.

Step 3: Counter progressive hardening of the arteries.

Now, let's go on to confront the challenges facing those who have experienced a ministroke.

Chapter Four

More on Ministrokes

Ellen, a sixty-two-year-old social worker, was going about her business one day when her body suddenly ceased to function properly. She found she could no longer talk correctly; she would think one word, and a completely different one—or a garbled sound—would come out. Not only that, she couldn't seem to feel objects well with the fingers of her right hand, and she had double vision.

At first, Ellen's colleagues thought she was joking. Then, they realized something serious had happened to her, and someone called the local emergency number for an ambulance. By the time the medics arrived, however, Ellen had returned to normal.

What had happened to Ellen? She had suffered a "ministroke," or transient ischemic attack (TIA). There was no permanent damage, but as already indicated, TIAs must always be taken *very* seriously as harbingers of full-fledged strokes.

Overcoming
the TIA Threat

Although about 10 percent of all strokes are preceded by a TIA, a ministroke is perhaps the best warning signal we have that a stroke is threatening. Within one year after experiencing a TIA, up to one half of patients will have a stroke. Furthermore, time is of the essence in assessing risk and responding medically.

What are the signals of a TIA? They include the following sudden transient symptoms:

* Motor impairment, such as an inability to use one or two limbs on the same side properly, or a lack of muscular coordination

* A loss or impairment of the senses, such as touch or taste

* Impairment of speech or inability to speak

* Double vision or varying degrees of blindness

* Visual difficulty in one eye

* An inability to understand, think, or reason clearly

* Dizziness

* Difficulty swallowing

* Memory loss

* Loss of consciousness

By definition, the symptoms accompanying a TIA are completely reversed within twenty-four hours. In fact, though, most ministrokes last only a few minutes and things are usually back to normal within one hour.

The medical response to a TIA. You may suspect it, but a physician must make the diagnosis that you have actually had a TIA. Consequently, it is essential for you to get to a doctor's office or hospital emergency room as quickly as possible.

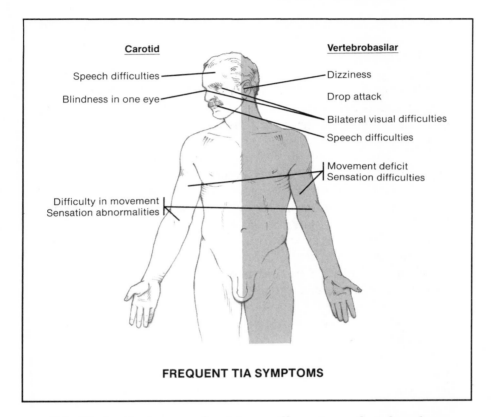

Carotid		Vertebrobasilar

Speech difficulties

Blindness in one eye

Dizziness

Drop attack

Bilateral visual difficulties

Speech difficulties

Movement deficit
Sensation difficulties

Difficulty in movement
Sensation abnormalities

FREQUENT TIA SYMPTOMS

It's likely that your physician will review what has happened and perform a physical examination. Further testing is likely. If your doctor concludes that you have had a TIA, he or she may prescribe a baby aspirin each day. (If you are allergic to aspirin, other medication will be substituted.) The theory is that aspirin can reduce the tendency of the blood to clot and thus may prevent tiny blockages in vessels that caused the TIA.

Most studies that have been conducted in different parts of the world support the benefits of aspirin in preventing stroke. Investigations here as well as in Holland, Germany, and France, for instance, have found use of aspirin to be associated with fewer strokes.

Although opinions regarding the appropriate dosage vary, one small "baby" aspirin (80 milligrams) per day would be appropriate for those who have had a TIA *or* for anyone who seems to have a higher than average risk for stroke or heart disease. Large doses of aspirin can be counterproductive and can be accompanied by gastrointestinal side effects.

A newly tested drug, ticlopidine, also shows promise. Recently approved by the Food and Drug Administration (FDA), this medication has been shown to be somewhat more effective than aspirin in reducing the risk of stroke in patients who have had a TIA. It is usually prescribed for those who cannot take aspirin. As with any medication, there are side effects, and cost may be a factor for some patients too. Check with your physician to see if this medication is appropriate for you.

Surgery is another possibility for those who have suffered a TIA. The most common procedure is called a carotid endarterectomy, which means scraping out the inner lining of the carotid artery in the neck. The purpose is to get rid of a clot or buildup of plaque in that artery. Otherwise, the clot may promote a blockage of blood to the brain or a traveling clot (embolus).

Past studies have been equivocal in supporting this procedure. Recent studies indicated that carotid endarterectomy was appropriate treatment in situations where 70 percent of the lumen (the inner, open part of the vessel's passageway) of the carotid artery was occluded (blocked).

___Is It Different from Dizziness?___

There has occasionally been some uncertainty about exactly what constitutes a TIA because some of the symptoms are the same or similar to those of other illnesses. In particular, a ministroke may become confused with dizziness or with fainting (syncope). In any event, fainting or syncope *doesn't necessarily* mean stroke.

Dizziness. Although dizziness, or vertigo, may be a symptom of a TIA, there are obviously many situations in which a person becomes dizzy without having a ministroke. Dizziness is a vague sort of problem that often occurs by itself, without other symptoms. At times, older patients may experience dizziness simply because their overall circulation is less efficient or more sluggish than that of younger people. Dizziness is a nonspecific complaint accompanying many disorders including ear problems and emotional problems.

Even young people who have been sitting for a while and then quickly stand up may experience the dizziness that accompanies too little blood flow to the brain. In such situations, the blood has pooled in the lower parts of the body and hasn't been given sufficient time to make it back to the head. Hyperventilation may also cause dizziness in both the young and old. So, clearly, there are many reasons for dizziness other than a TIA!

Dizziness may also precede the fainting that characterizes syncope, which in many ways is much closer to a TIA than are these other conditions.

The syncope scenario. Syncope, or fainting, is defined as a temporary loss of consciousness. This phenomenon occurs when the circulation to the brain is temporarily interrupted for an estimated eight to ten seconds. A stroke, on the other hand, is a disability resulting from the death of nerve cells in the brain, which results from the prolonged deprivation of cerebral blood flow. A TIA is somewhere in the middle. The brain is deprived of blood longer with a TIA than with syncope—hence, the more serious, strokelike symptoms that accompany the TIA, or ministroke. On the other hand, the TIA falls far short of a full stroke because the symptoms are temporary, and the body quickly returns to normal.

Since the circulation to the brain is affected in all three of these problems, they have a common feature. But the terms may become confused if we don't keep the precise understanding of each condition in mind.

To get a better grasp on syncope, it is instructive to take a page from the novels of the Victorian era, in which ladies often "swooned." This literary motif eventually faded and was replaced by straightforward fainting episodes in some of today's romance literature (or, for that matter, in some television drama and comedy). Whatever the era, the literary swoon or faint usually has resulted from an emotional crisis. But in the real world, there may be other factors that trigger syncope or fainting.

To begin with, physicians consider any fainting or syncope a significant medical event. Sometimes the condition isn't serious, but frequently it is. At all times, the symptom requires close medical evaluation. To understand how syncope may occur, consider the following actual case illustrations.

Case 1: Tom C. was a fifty-year-old railroad engineer whose uniform was well fitted and pressed, from his firm starched collar down to spit-shined shoes. But he had a problem. He would regularly black out when his train went around a sharp bend.

An examination revealed that Tom had "carotid sinus hypersensitivity." Explanation: The carotid sinus is an anatomical site in the major neck artery that helps control heart rate and blood pressure. When Tom turned his head sharply as the train turned, his firm neck collar compressed his carotid sinus, thus causing a lowering of the blood pressure and slowing of the heart. Syncope resulted, and Tom "blacked out" momentarily.

The solution: Tom wore open-collared shirts and took medication to counter the problem.

Case 2: Richard B. is a thirty-one-year-old attorney who had dinner at a roadside café. The next morning he suffered severe abdominal pain. In the midst of this attack, he went to the bathroom, fainted, and suffered a laceration of his scalp.

Explanation: This is an example of "reflex syncope," or "situational syncope." Automatic reflex systems in the body cause a lowering of blood pressure and heart rate and a temporary decrease in blood flowing to the brain. Richard's intense abdominal pain initiated reflexes that caused fainting. Similar symptoms may occur in people who have paroxysms of coughing (ptussic syncope), or who are in the act of voiding (micturation syncope), or who are having a bowel movement (defecation syncope), or who are swallowing (deglutition syncope).

Case 3: Charles C. is a nineteen-year-old military cadet who is well motivated and loves his profession. While standing at attention during a parade, however, he fainted.

Explanation: When a person stands for a long period fairly rigidly in one place, blood pools in the lower extremities and the lower part of the body. Blood is ordinarily propelled toward the heart by the action of the muscles of the lower extremities.

Charles stood at attention absolutely motionless. Insufficient blood was thus pushed toward his heart, and the result was a drop in blood pressure. He recovered promptly and now has learned to move his legs ever so slightly, even when standing at attention.

"Orthostatic syncope" is a term that simply means that the blood pressure falls instead of rising. Many people experience this syncope when they arise quickly from a sitting position to answer a doorbell or a telephone.

Case 4: Edmund C., who was forty-two years of age, was confined to bed for several days because of a fever. Upon recovering, he hopped out of bed and fainted.

Explanation: Prolonged bed rest can lead to deconditioning of the muscles of the body and a lowering of blood pressure. Assuming an upright posture suddenly caused Edmund to have syncope because he could not maintain adequate blood pressure and blood flow to the brain. Prolonged bed rest can also result in the far more serious pulmonary embolus—a traveling clot to the lung.

Case 5: James W., nine years old, fainted in school and experienced movements in his arms and legs, according to a report by his teacher.

Explanation: James had a seizure owing to an irritable area in the brain. In effect, he had an epileptic attack. He is now taking medications that enable him to engage in full activities. He is now in good health.

The more serious types of syncope generally occur in the older age groups. Cerebral blood flow decreases with aging, and syncope may be the first manifestation of various serious illnesses, including heart disease, in the elderly. Here are some illustrations:

Case 6: Bess W. is a seventy-two-year-old who fainted several times after eating.

Explanation: One of Bess's heart valves had thickened and narrowed over the years (a process called aortic stenosis). When Bess ate a large meal, blood was diverted to her stomach, thus depriving her brain of circulation. Fortunately, Bess was able to have her valve replaced. She now functions quite well, without any fainting episodes.

Case 7: Eustace R. is a sixty-year-old accountant who was on his way to the store to replenish his supply of cigarettes. He suffered squeezing chest pain and fainted.

Explanation: Eustace's chest pain was caused by a heart attack, precipitated in part by smoking, a high-fat diet, and high blood pressure. His heart was temporarily unable to pump sufficient blood to the brain. The "fainting spell" was really syncope due to a heart attack.

Case 8: Elvira C. is a vibrant seventy-eight-year-old who suffered several fainting spells over a period of two weeks before consulting her physician. She had always been in good health, but she noticed an occasional "skipped beat" of the heart and wondered if this was related to her fainting spells.

Explanation: Elvira had suffered a condition known as heart block. She did not have a heart attack, but she did have an abnormal, irregular heartbeat. Instead of the usual sixty'eighty beats per minute, her heartbeat was recorded as thirty-four beats per minute. A pacemaker was inserted to correct the abnormality.

More than fifty thousand new cases of heart block occur annually in the United States. It is estimated that half of these people experience syncope before the condition is detected.

First-line examination for syncope. If you have suffered a fainting spell, your physician will want to know your personal health history and any prescribed medications you're taking. Sometimes, drugs can cause syncope. Your physician will also determine your blood pressure in the sitting and standing positions. In addition, he or she will check your neck pulse and listen to the action of your heart.

The exam will include an evaluation of your nervous system, and a testing of your strength, sensation ability, and reflexes.

CAUSES OF TIA (TRANSIENT ISCHEMIA ATTACK OR "MINI STROKES")
ATHERO SCLERASIS OF ARTERIES GOING TO THE BRAIN

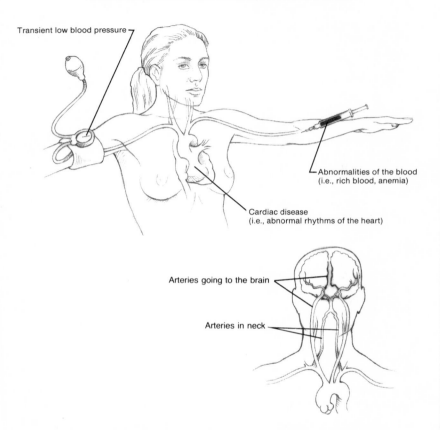

Transient low blood pressure

Abnormalities of the blood
(i.e., rich blood, anemia)

Cardiac disease
(i.e., abnormal rhythms of the heart)

Arteries going to the brain

Arteries in neck

ATHEROSCLEROSIS OF ARTERIES GOING TO THE BRAIN

Table 2. Causes of Fainting

Abnormalities of Circulatory Control

Diuretics, hemorrhage, diarrhea, dehydration
Vasodilators (nitrates and calcium channel blockers)
Autonomic
Reflex causes
Carotid sinus hypersensitivity

Abnormalities of Cardiac Function

Inadequate filling of heart
Disease of heart valves and heart muscle
Cardiac arrhythmias (abnormal cardiac rhythm)
Bradycardias (heart rate too slow)
Tachycardias (heart rate too fast)

Metabolic Disturbances

Hypoglycemia (low blood sugar)
Hypocapnia (hyperventilation)
Intoxication (alcohol, drugs)

Neurologic Causes

Seizures
Cerebrovascular disease
Intracranial hemorrhage
Tumors (of brain)
Hysteria (swooning)

Also, you will undergo a blood test, an electroencephalogram (EEG), and an electrocardiogram (ECG). Pinpointing the cause of your syncope through such tests is important because appropriate treatment is available and usually quite effective.

Finally, it is important to keep in mind the distinction between syncope on the one hand, and TIAs and strokes on the other. Syncope may certainly be a serious signal of a health problem, but it's not usually linked to stroke. Furthermore, a ministroke, or TIA, rarely causes fainting episodes—though a TIA may be accompanied by sudden drop attacks (falling to the floor while still conscious) because of the onset of weakness in both legs.

If a fainting spell occurs, you should definitely see a physician. But don't worry that you're on the verge of a stroke, because you probably are not. A TIA, not syncope, is the preliminary event that will place you at risk for stroke. In any case, the one thing that a fainting spell and a TIA have in common is the need for prompt evaluation by your physician.

Chapter Five

Meet High Blood Pressure Head-on

Hypertension—or sustained high blood pressure—may occur in very young people, but in most cases it is considered a midlife disease. What's the definition of "midlife"? The best way to answer this question is to think in terms of the *effects* of aging, rather than a specific range of years. So if you have some of the signs of middle age—bulges, bagginess, balding, white or graying hair, or bad vision—then you're more likely to confront problems with high blood pressure.

To understand why it is so important to meet high blood pressure *head-on*—and lower those readings before it's too late—consider these two very different scenarios:

Scenario 1: Ryan T., fifty-seven years old, was admitted to a hospital emergency room after suffering a cerebral hemorrhage, or bleeding in the brain. He was unable to speak or use the right side of his body. The process of recovery was slow and incomplete.

Although the stroke occurred swiftly and unexpectedly, the groundwork for this tragedy had been laid more than twenty years before, when Ryan's blood pressure first began to rise. When he was only thirty-five, his blood pressure was measured as a high normal 138/88. Readings of 120/80 are considered normal, while those of 140/90 or above are considered high—hence the term "high blood pressure," or hypertension. Within two years, his measurements had risen to an average of 143/92, which is in the mild hypertensive range.

In the ensuing years, Ryan's blood pressure crept up, primarily for two reasons. First, he failed to take his physician's advice to lose weight, cut back on alcohol consumption, and reduce his intake of salty foods. In other words, he didn't take seriously the importance of changing his life-style in ways that would help reduce or at least control his high readings.

Second, Ryan neglected to take regularly the medications that his physician recommended. After his average blood pressure readings had risen above about 160/95, diuretics had been prescribed. But Ryan felt uncomfortable because they caused him to urinate frequently and thus disturbed his sleep. He also experienced a decrease in sexual functioning. Because of these problems, he often didn't take his medicine and eventually stopped entirely. There was a resultant rise in his blood pressure.

On a couple of occasions, Ryan's physician tried other medications, such as the "beta-blockers." But Ryan felt this type of medication slowed him down too much and also contributed to his sexual impairment. In fact, the problem at this stage may have been partially psychological: Ryan may have lacked confidence that he could perform adequately sexually with *any* antihypertensive drug. So he may have experienced some amount of ongoing impotence simply because he *believed* he would be impotent with medications.

Finally, when he was in his mid-fifties, Ryan's blood pressure was hovering in the neighborhood of 170/100. His physician persuaded him at long last to become more faithful with his medications, in part because he had switched to a drug with fewer side effects, the new ACE inhibitors. These medications have developed a reputation for creating fewer side effects, including sexual problems. Ryan came to believe that the drug would work for him as well. Indeed, he did quite well. His blood pressure declined to normal levels, and he had increased feelings of well-being.

Unfortunately, Ryan went out of town on a three-week business trip and forgot to take along his high blood pressure medicine. He felt relatively well—up until the moment of his stroke. It hit like a bolt from the blue, completely without warning.

For about twenty years, Ryan had failed to control his hypertension, and his final effort to be careful had come too late. This neglect had resulted in damage to the arteries throughout his body, but particularly those in his brain. A weak spot in the wall of one of those vessels finally ruptured, blood spilled into the brain, and a stroke ensued.

Ryan will undoubtedly recover to some extent from the damage done to his brain. But he will probably always have some disability as a result of his stroke.

Scenario 2: Like Ryan, Sandy discovered when she was in her mid-thirties that her blood pressure was too high. Her measurements were actually somewhat worse than Ryan's: She had a reading of 140/95 when she was checked at age thirty-four—a level that placed her at the outset of the mild hypertension category.

Because Sandy's blood pressure was still in the mild or borderline range, her physician made recommendations that were similar to those Ryan had received about altering her life-style. Among other things, she was told to stop smoking, lose the fifteen pounds of extra weight she was carrying, exercise more regularly, and cut back on salty foods.

She thought all this was a tall order because when she stopped smoking, she usually gained weight. But through personal commitment and hard work, she increased her exercise routine, stopped smoking—and managed not to gain weight. She credited the increased exercise with being responsible for her better weight control. In the end, Sandy managed, without medications, to bring her blood pressure back into the high normal range, around 135/86.

After about fifteen years, however, the readings crept up again into the mild hypertension range. At that time, her doctor placed her on medications similar to those that had been prescribed for Ryan. Sandy was quite conscientious about taking her medication, and as a result, her blood pressure remained well within the normal range.

Sandy, at fifty-nine years of age, is now two years older than Ryan. But she enjoys good health, and her risk for stroke is not much higher than anyone else's.

It is important to understand how the wise management of high blood pressure has almost certainly given Sandy a healthier and longer lease on life than Ryan. To that end, I want to pose and answer four key action questions that will enhance your understanding of the threat of hypertension.

Question 1: What's the Link Between High ____Blood Pressure and Stroke?____

There are two basic ways that high blood pressure may be linked to stroke. The first involves steady weakening of the vessel walls, while the second focuses more on accelerating the process of hardening the walls of the arteries.

Weakening the walls. A significant increase in blood pressure is likely to encourage a weakening and ballooning of the vessel walls in the brain. Too much such pressure over too long a period of time will make the vessel walls more vulnerable to rupture. Ruptures in the vessel wall will allow the blood to flow out into the brain tissue and cause serious damage. This is what happened with Ryan's stroke.

Damage to the walls. High blood pressure over a period of time may also cause defects in the inner vessel lining. These rough and damaged areas promote collecting of plaque, the fatty deposits consisting of cholesterol and fats. Again, the duration and degree of blood pressure elevation are usually the factors that determine how much damage is done to the arteries and the extent to which they are predisposed to blockage. Those who have suffered from the problem of hypertension for years become more vulnerable to a stroke resulting from an obstruction to blood vessels leading to the brain.

These vessel-blocking, or thrombotic, types of strokes occur when a clot develops in vessels that have been narrowed by the buildup of obstructive plaque. The clogging reduces the flow of blood to the brain tissue, and the affected part of the brain is injured and may die.

To guard against these two threats to the brain—the weakening and damaging of the vessel walls—it is important first to know what your blood pressure is. Then you will be in a better position to take steps to keep it normal.

Question 2:
What's High, What's Low—
_____and How Can I Know?_____

The blood vessels are a closed system of constricting and dilating tubes that carry blood from the heart, to the tissues, and back to the heart. Specifically, *arteries* carry blood from the heart to the tissues of the body; *veins* carry it to the heart from the tissues; and *capillaries* are intermediary connections between arteries and veins. Blood flows through the vessels primarily because of the motion imparted to it by the pumping of the heart.

As a pump, the heart has two main purposes: (1) It must propel enough blood throughout the body to assure an adequate flow of the oxygen and nutrients carried by the blood to all body tissues. And (2) it must also provide the power to remove carbon dioxide and waste products from those tissues. Blood pressure is simply the amount of pressure the heart requires to pump the blood from the heart throughout the body. It is measured in terms of millimeters of mercury.

Blood pressure, by the way, is not unique to human beings; any animal with a heart pumps blood through its circulatory system. The blood pressure varies depending on the species. Animals with the longest necks have the highest pressures because more force is needed to get blood up into the brain from the heart. The normal pressure of a giraffe, for example, is well over twice as high as that of a human. Birds have higher blood pressure than mammals because their pressure has to overcome gravity as well as the accelerating and decelerating forces common to flying.

As for the human heart, that organ has its own distinctive features. The average adult human heart is normally only about the size of a clenched fist—but no pump of any size devised by man can outperform it. One has to stand in respectful awe of any pump that, in the average person, can put out 500 million quarts of blood over a seventy-year period. This estimate, by the way, is based on the heart at rest. It doesn't take into account exercise or stress that increases the flow—and the pressure.

Blood pressure depends not only on the heart pump, but also on the state of the tubes (arteries, veins, and capillaries) through which the blood flows. If the diameter of the vessel tube is narrowed, we speak of an increased resistance. If the vessel's diameter is increased, the resistance is decreased. In high blood pressure there is usually an increase in resistance to the flow of blood.

Blood pressure, then, is determined both by the amount of blood pumped by the heart and by the resistance that the blood encounters in flowing through the vessels.

How Blood Pressure Is Measured

When the heart beats, it first contracts. With this act, the heart pressure increases in order to pump out the blood through the arteries. Then it relaxes to allow blood to flow back into the heart. The contraction phase is known as the *systole,* and the relaxation phase is the *diastole.* Thus, *systolic blood pressure* is the top pressure reached when the heart contracts or gets smaller (clenches tightly). The *diastolic blood pressure* is the lowest pressure reached when the heart relaxes.

In recording blood pressure, the systolic reading is written over the diastolic, and the measurements are given in millimeters of mercury, or mm Hg. So normal blood pressure would be written as 120/80 mm Hg, or just 120/80 (read as "one twenty over eighty"). This means that the systolic pressure is 120, and the diastolic pressure is 80.

The apparatus customarily used to measure blood pressure is the sphygmomanometer—which may be a mouthful to say, but is a common sight in any doctor's office. This device consists of an inflatable cuff that is placed around the arm and a gauge, which is used with a stethoscope. Nowadays, though, many automatic machines are available with a microphone and a digital readout screen.

After the cuff is placed around the upper arm, it is pumped up to stop the flow of arterial blood for a few moments. Then the person taking the reading reduces pressure in the cuff. At the same time, one listens through a stethoscope, which is placed on the artery just below the cuff. (Note: No stethoscope is attached to the electronic blood pressure devices.) The blood pressure is usually recorded in the supine or lying-down position, sitting or standing positions.

As the person taking the measurement listens, he will hear a tap-tap-tapping sound that signals the arterial flow is beginning again beneath the loosened cuff. The point on the pressure gauge at which the first tap is heard corresponds to the systolic pressure. As the cuff is further deflated, the tapping sounds eventually disappear. The point at which the sounds stop is the marker for the diastolic pressure.

Why Blood Pressure Readings Change

Blood pressure may vary for any number of reasons, which may have little to do with high blood pressure. One factor may be the sphygmomanometer itself. Though the device is basically quite simple, the cuff must be the correct size to get accurate readings. A too-wide cuff will give false readings, as will a too-narrow one. In fact, it is not unusual to get false high readings in obese people because the cuff is too narrow. (Also, as we'll see shortly, obesity is related to elevation of blood pressure.)

The blood pressure in young healthy adults in the sitting or lying position at rest is approximately 120/80. Since the blood pressure is the product of the amount of blood pumped by the heart and the resistance to flow in the arteries, it is affected by conditions related to both of those factors. Emotional factors, for example, increase the heart's output and will cause an increased blood pressure in many excited or tense individuals. Conversely, emotional or physical relaxation will lower the pressure. Other activities that may increase blood pressure include exercise, bowel and bladder functions, and sexual activities.

The time of day is another factor that may affect blood pressure. In particular, systolic blood pressure varies considerably throughout the day. It is usually relatively low during sleep but rises abruptly between 8:00 A.M. and 11:00 A.M. Then the pressure tends to fall in the afternoon, though it may rise dramatically during periods of stress or exercise. There is considerable variation in the blood pressure in the course of our daily activities. That is normal.

In healthy humans, both the systolic and diastolic pressures rise with age. Generally speaking, the systolic pressure increase is greater than the diastolic. A significant cause of the rise of systolic pressure is the decreased elasticity of the arteries as their walls become more rigid with advancing age. With older people, systolic blood pressure tends to increase by about 1 millimeter of mercury a year. Diastolic blood pressure goes up by about 0.4 mm Hg a year. Hormonal changes may account for other changes in blood pressure. For example, women from age forty to fifty tend to have lower blood pressure than women over fifty or than men of any age.

What about the effect of exercise? A normal response to rigorous physical activity is an increase in blood pressure. Systolic pressure rises initially, and this increase is followed by a fall in diastolic pressure. Paradoxically, although exercise places an extra requirement on the heart, it also is one of the most powerful stimuli to *relax* blood vessels and decrease vessel resistance.

In short, exercise programs often help *lower* blood pressure in the long run, even though pressure may go up temporarily during a workout. Other conditions that have had an impact on blood pressure include race and socioeconomic circumstances. Blacks have generally higher blood pressures than whites. Similarly, the Japanese in Japan tend to have higher pressures than the Japanese in Hawaii or in the mainland United States.

What accounts for these differences? Diet is one possibility. Many blacks and Japanese (in Japan), for instance, have a relatively high salt intake in their diets. The groups with higher blood pressures tend to consume more salt than other groups. Also, genetics may play a role in the variations among different ethnic groups.

Another interesting factor that may raise blood pressure is a phenomenon known as "white coat hypertension." This condition refers to the fact that many people to some extent experience a rise in blood pressure just by anticipating having their blood pressure readings taken. When they see a person with a white coat who is holding a blood pressure machine, their pressure begins to climb! To guard against this problem and other variables, two or three readings should be taken during the medical exam. The pressures of most people will decline into their true range after they have become more comfortable with their surroundings.

Others, however, may continue to experience high blood pressure readings while they are in the doctor's office, even though outside the office, their blood pressure is normal. Indeed there are patients whose blood pressure readings are higher when the measurement is taken by a physician than when it is taken by a nurse. In these situations, monitoring of the blood pressure at home, as well as twenty-four-hour electronic monitoring, are being used to distinguish white coat hypertension from true hypertension. Home blood pressure measuring devices are available. They can be used to help distinguish those who need treatment for hypertension from those who don't and as a guide to the effectiveness of therapy.

High Versus Normal Blood Pressure

High blood pressure, or hypertension, has been recognized as a disease only since the turn of the twentieth century, when the sphygmomanometer was invented. But it has been hard over the years to define what is a "normal" or a "high" measurement. For example, a "normal" blood pressure of slightly less than 140/90 may be normal for adults, but is *not* normal for children. According to the Joint National Committee on Detection, Evaluation, and Treatment of High Blood Pressure, the upper limits of normal for a child under six years of age should be 110/75.

The current consensus is that normal blood pressure for adults should be less than 140/90. Mild diastolic hypertension is in the 90–104 range. Moderate diastolic hypertension is 105–114 mm Hg. And severe diastolic hypertension is a reading of 115 or above. Borderline systolic hypertension is 140–159. Full-blown systolic hypertension is 160 or above.

The Joint National Committee on Detection, Evaluation, and Treatment of High Blood Pressure has stated its official policy this way: "The diagnosis of hypertension in adults is confirmed when the average of two or more diastolic blood pressures on at least two subsequent visits is 90 mm Hg or higher or when the average of multiple systolic blood pressures on 2 or more subsequent visits is consistently greater than 140 mm Hg" (from "The 1988 Report of the Joint National Committee on Detection, Evaluation, and Treatment of High Blood Pressure").

Question 3: What Factors Put Me at Risk for _____High Blood Pressure?_____

We have already discussed in some detail in Chapters Three and Four the risk factors that may predispose a person to stroke. Among other things, we learned that having high blood pressure, or hypertension, is a major reason that many people suffer a stroke and/or a heart attack.

Now, let's delve into this issue of high blood pressure a little more deeply. Obviously, if you can head off hypertension, you may also be able to head off a stroke. So the pressing question now becomes, What factors currently in my life place me at risk for high blood pressure—and what can I do about them? In the following discussion, I have identified eight main factors that may put you at greater risk for high blood pressure hypertension, and hence for stroke. In each case, there's an indication of the extent to which you can change or modify those factors and thus lower your risk. Some of these have already been mentioned as general risk factors for stroke in Chapter Three. But I believe it's also important to reiterate them here as risk factors specific to high blood pressure, which is such an important precondition for many strokes.

Factor 1: A previous high blood pressure measurement. A person who has had one high blood pressure reading at some point in the past is statistically at a higher risk of developing high blood pressure later than a person who has never had such a reading. Still, not everyone with a high blood pressure reading necessarily has high blood pressure disease. About 60 million people have had at least one high blood pressure measurement. But of those individuals, only about 40 million have repeat high readings that justify classifying them as hypertensive patients.

In any event, it is extremely important to ascertain your precise blood pressure status with more than one reading. Hypertension is responsible for about 10–15 percent of deaths in people over fifty years of age. Insurance studies reveal that at age forty-five, a systolic pressure above 150 mm Hg will reduce life expectancy of men by 11.5 years and women by 8.5 years.

Two or three readings done when a person is at rest in a relaxed atmosphere should be sufficient to determine who really does have or does not have a significantly elevated blood pressure.

Factor 2: Advancing age. The older you get, the more likely it is that your blood pressure will rise. For that reason, a rough rule of thumb developed years ago in the medical community says that you can expect your systolic blood pressure to be as high as 100 plus your age. For example, if you're fifty, your systolic pressure would be 150. However, a systolic blood pressure over 150 at any age is considered too high.

This rule of thumb should be accepted *only* as an outside upper limit, however. If you maintain a healthy life-style designed to prevent the onset of high blood pressure, you can keep your measurements lower than those of most people your age. Still, some rise can be expected with increasing years.

Factor 3: A family history of hypertension. Your chances of having high blood pressure are double those of the average person if one of your parents had this health problem. Your risk is also greater if a brother or sister has the disease. A tendency toward high blood pressure may also be genetic.

The incidence of hypertension is higher in blacks than in whites at every age. While 10 white men in 100,000 die of hypertension annually, 66 black men are so affected. Furthermore, four times as many black women as white women have the disease.

Hypertension is especially dangerous to older blacks. Half of blacks over age sixty-five have high blood pressure, according to the National Institutes of Health. In contrast, two out of five whites that age have a problem with hypertension. We need to depend on the results of research to tell us why race is such an important factor. Obviously, there's nothing you can do to change your family or ethnic heritage. On the other hand, you can minimize the impact of any inherited tendency by changing negative features in your life-style, such as obesity, smoking, excess salt use, alcohol abuse, and high cholesterol—all of which are described in greater detail below.

Factor 4: Obesity. Carrying around excess weight can contribute significantly to high blood pressure. In the Framingham study, for instance, participants who were 20 percent or more above their best weight were *eight times* more likely than less obese people to develop high blood pressure!

Another consideration with weight is the location of the fatty tissue. Excess fat around the abdomen and chest has been linked to hypertension more often than fat around the buttocks, hips, and upper legs.

Sophisticated studies on eating disorders and obesity are in progress. Chemical and mechanical receptors in the stomach and small intestine are thought to send signals to stop eating. Elucidation of obesity remains a research problem.

In the meanwhile, until we know more, we must rely on eating less and exercising more. Overall weight reduction will almost always result in lowering the blood pressure.

Factor 5: Alcohol abuse. Large population surveys have shown that drinking more than two ounces of alcohol a day (as contained in four beers or four glasses of wine or four mixed drinks) is linked to higher blood pressure. Hypertension expert Dr. Norman Kaplan of the University of Texas Southwestern Medical School in Dallas observes further that more than three ounces a day (six beers, six glasses of wine, or six mixed drinks) has been associated with full-blown hypertension.

Obviously, this is an important *controllable* risk factor for hypertension. So evaluate your drinking habits. If you drink, limit your alcohol intake to no more than two beers, two glasses of wine, or two mixed drinks daily.

Factor 6: *A negative response to salt.* As many as 50 percent of all those with high blood pressure experience a negative response to the salt in their diets. In other words, the more salt they consume, the higher their blood pressure measurements become. Various scientific studies have helped establish that the salt connection is the most solid link between nutrition and blood pressure. In the 1940s, for example, high blood pressure was successfully reduced without medication by the Kempner diet, which consisted of rice, fruit, and sugar. This has a very low sodium content.

In other experiments, animals have been selectively bred to develop hypertension when they were fed salt. On a low-salt diet, these salt-sensitive animals have normal blood pressure. When their salt intake is raised, the sensitive animals retain the salt and develop hypertension. In contrast, salt-*resistant* animals that are tested excrete the additional sodium, and their blood pressure remains normal.

A survey of various "primitive" societies around the world also reveals some interesting facts about hypertension and salt consumption. Populations with low salt intake in Africa, Australia, New Guinea, Brazil, and Venezuela have low incidence of high blood pressure. When those societies become "developed" or "civilized," however, the result is urbanization, psychological stress, decreased physical activity, and increased salt consumption. Rises in blood pressure soon follow. So the "civilized" way of life may well be the salt-rich and hypertensive way of life!

In an anthropological commentary, S. Boyd Eaton and his colleagues at Emory University in Atlanta point out that while human genetic makeup has not appreciably changed during the past ten thousand years, we are now subject to "disease of civilization." Some "primitive societies" surviving to the present day, resemble humans of the late Paleolithic period (20,000 to 35,000 years ago) with respect to diet and exercise. New Guinea highland natives, Solomon Islanders, and Kalahari San (Bushmen) are some of the groups in which high blood pressure and high cholesterol are extremely rare. Their lives are characterized by very low fat intake and considerable physical exercise. Serum cholesterol values in most groups were found to be under 150 milligrams. Obesity and diabetes were virtually absent in these "primitive" peoples.

How can you determine whether you are sensitive to salt or not? It's hard, and to be precise, extensive and expensive tests would have to be conducted. So most hypertensive patients, as well as those thought to be at risk for high blood pressure, are just advised to go on a low-salt diet. This regimen certainly can't hurt, and it will definitely lower anyone's risk for hypertension.

How low is low when you are designing a low-salt diet? It is estimated that the average American takes in the prodigious pile of about ten grams of salt daily. That amount can be translated into 2½ teaspoons of salt per day—far too much for anyone. Many low-salt diets are designed to cut in half this commonly consumed amount. In other words, the recommendation is to eat only a total of five grams or less of salt each day.

Many practical problems face those who want to try the low-salt route. First of all, salt content and sodium content must be distinguished. The content of sodium on food labels is often given in milligrams or equivalent measurements. The sodium component of salt, which makes up about 40 percent of the product (chloride accounts for the other 60 percent), is thought to be the main culprit in hypertension. So, many authorities talk in terms of sodium rather than salt. But the problem is that the ordinary person does not carry around a sodium table and a calculator.

Here's a quick way to calculate the sodium content of salt: Multiply the amount of salt by ⅖ (or by.4 if you prefer to use decimals) to get the amount of sodium. Sodium is measured in milligrams (mg) or grams (g); 1,000 milligrams equal 1 gram. One teaspoon of salt weighs 4 grams (or 4,000 milligrams) and thus contains 1,600 milligrams of sodium. Using this simple formula, you would find that the average daily consumption by Americans of 10 grams of salt would translate to 4 grams of sodium. Also, a low-*sodium* diet would involve 5 grams of salt or 2 grams or less of sodium daily (⅖ or .4 times 5 grams of salt).

Note: There is "hidden" salt in virtually everything you eat or drink. Even tapwater has small amounts of sodium chloride (salt). Most canned foods contain unnecessarily large amounts of salt. Salt is used as a preservative as well as a flavoring agent by manufacturers. Pickled, cured, and smoked foods are processed with and likewise contain excessive amounts of salt. The amount of sodium our body needs is only about 250 to 500 milligrams per day.

Mothers may even add salt to their babies' formula, ostensibly to stimulate the child's appetite. Yet babies' taste buds do not mature till about two years of age!

Here are some simple guidelines to help you keep your salt intake low:

* Milk, cheese, bread, and cereals are rich sources of sodium. Fruits and potatoes are relatively low in sodium. Processed and preserved foods introduce large amounts of sodium.

* Never use table salt on your food.

* Substitute other flavorings and spices in cooking to provide adequate taste and desirable flavor. Ginger, oregano, pepper, chili powder, garlic, onion powder, paprika, curry, parsley, and basil are among the food flavors that don't contain salt.

    On average, 20 percent of dietary sodium is naturally present in the food, almost 50 percent is added in food processing, and 30 percent is added by the consumer. So hide the salt shaker! Use the other seasoning agents listed above; they contain no salt and can add flavor to almost any meal.

* Salt-rich foods should be avoided like the plague. Bacon, hot dogs, canned soups, sausages, potato chips, pretzels, ketchup, and fast-food burgers are all rich in salt. Usually, when you cut back on these foods, the taste buds

become more sensitive to salt, and the appetite for salt declines after a few months.

* Check the labels on foods you buy. Select the low-salt or no-salt varieties, and *always* check the number of grams or milligrams of salt or sodium contained in the food. Granted, you'll have to do some simple mathematics for several representative days of meals to see how much salt you're consuming. But these easy calculations will give you a much better idea of how you can restrict your intake.

* For those foods that don't come with labels, such as meats or poultry, buy a book like the *Handbook of the Nutritional Contents of Foods,* published by the United States Department of Agriculture. There, for example, you'll learn that the average sodium value per 100 grams (3.5 ounces) of all cuts of beef is 370 milligrams for cooked meat.

For your reference, I have included Table 3 showing the approximate hidden sodium content, in millequivalents (mEq), in various foods. Fortunately, current regulations now call for labeling the sodium content of foods.

Table 3.   Approximate Sodium Content of Selected Foods

Foods by Group	Approx. Portion	Approx. Sodium (mEq)
Meat		
Unsalted	1 oz	1
Salted	1 oz	3
Cottage cheese (dry curd)	1/4 cup	1
Egg	1 med	3
Mild aged cheddar cheese	1 oz	8
Cottage cheese, creamed	1/4 cup	10

Foods by Group	Approx. Portion	Approx. Sodium (mEq)
Ham	1 oz	12–18
Processed American cheese food	1 oz	12–15
Cold cuts	1 oz	14–18
Smoked link sausage	1 oz	18
Milk		
Whole	8 oz	5
Skim, nonfat, or 1%	8 oz	6
Buttermilk (from skim milk)	8 oz	14
Starch		
Puffed ready-to-eat cereal	1½ cups	0–1.5
Low sodium bread	1 slice	0.5
Cooked potatoes, cereals, and other starches (unsalted) (pasta, rice, etc.)	1/2 cup	0.5
Salt-free soda crackers	six 2″ sq	6
Graham crackers	three 2½″ sq	6
Regular bread	1 slice	5
Regular saltine crackers	six 2″ sq	11
Cooked potatoes, cereals, and other starches (salted)	1/2 cup	10
Corn or wheat flake cold cereal	3/4 cup	10
Pancake, biscuit, waffle (from mix)	1 med	10–15
Commercial soup	1 cup	15–40
Vegetables		
Unsalted (most kinds)	1/2 cup	Trace–1
Raw celery	3 stalks	3
Reg. canned (except tomatoes)	1/2 cup	10

Foods by Group	Approx. Portion	Approx. Sodium (mEq)
Reg. canned tomatoes, sauce or puree	1/4 cup	7–12
Reg. canned tomato juice	1/2 cup	19
Reg. vegetable juice cocktail	1/2 cup	19
Dill pickle	1 med	62
Fruit		
Most kinds, fruit or juice	1/2 cup	Trace
Fat		
Cream (any weight)	1 Tbsp	Trace
Vegetable oil	1 tsp	Trace
Unsalted butter, margarine	1 tsp	Trace
Regular mayonnaise	1 tsp	1
Regular butter, margarine	1 tsp	2
Mayonnaise type salad dressing	2 tsp	3
Green olives	9–10 small	27–30
Regular pourable salad dressing (average)	1 Tbsp	7
Blue cheese salad dressing	1 Tbsp	6–11
Bacon	1 med strip	7
Commercial gravy or gravy mix	2 Tbsp	7
Tartar sauce	1½ tsp	4

NOTE: Reprinted, by permission, from the *Mayo Clinic Diet Manual*, "Nutritional Management of Diseases and Disorders," p. 77).

Factor 7: A lack of exercise. As I have already indicated, it might seem that exercise is *bad* for those with mild hypertension. But that is not so. In fact, blood pressure rises during exercise in hypertensive patients more than it does in those with normal blood pressure.

Vigorous activity does increase the heart's output of blood, and the greater blood volume pushes harder against the vessel walls. The result is a rise in blood pressure, which can be documented with a blood pressure device during the exercise or any stress test. But the blood pressure levels return to normal more slowly among those with high blood pressure than among normal people.

A regular physical training program can actually *change* the body's control of blood pressure. Various studies have shown that those with mild elevations in blood pressure—say in the range of 140/90 to 159/94—can experience a permanent reduction in blood pressure levels. Many have actually achieved normal readings as a result of regular, though moderate, endurance-type exercise, such as walking briskly for a couple of miles, three to four times a week.

Caution: Not all exercises are good for people with high blood pressure. For example, isometric exercises, such as weightlifting or movements involving strenuous pushing or pulling, should be avoided.

Having offered these caveats, however, I want to return to my basic point: Embarking on an intelligent, easy endurance exercise program is something that can provide benefits to almost anyone. Start out modestly and gradually increase the exercise. Too much, too fast, too soon, and it will be too bad.

Dr. George Sheehan has written extensively about the mystical joys and practical benefits of exercise.

And remember: The more life-style changes you make in such areas as your physical activity, weight level, and drinking habits, the more you will be able to minimize the impact of genetic influences or other factors you thought you couldn't change.

Factor 8: Emotional disturbances. Many people experience "spikes," or sharp rises in their blood pressure levels, when they are confronted with stressful situations, such as a job crisis or a family difficulty.

For example, a number of studies have found that patients with high blood pressure have trouble acknowledging their angry feelings and are less likely than people with normal pressure to express their anger overtly.* One conclusion of some researchers is that suppressed hostility may have as great an effect on blood pressure as any of the other more commonly recognized risk factors.

Current evidence does not support the concept that the so-called type A personality (a competitive, aggressive, impatient individual) is more likely to get a stroke or heart attack. Stressful life events, such as bereavement owing to the death of a loved one, are more likely to be associated with cardiovascular disease.

How can you limit the impact of the emotional factors in your life? Here are some suggestions:

* As much as possible, avoid stressful situations and people. It's not always possible to run away from the circumstances that are triggering unhealthy increases in blood pressure. But the more you can limit your exposure to these influences, the better off you'll be.

* People who tend to suppress their anger should learn to be more assertive and to express their anger instead. The idea is not simply to explode. Rather, it is important to overcome habits of excessive submissiveness or reserve and to learn to confront in a rational fashion those people and situations that are the source of anger.

* Feelings of worry and anxiety can often be reduced with relaxation techniques. One of the most commonly used concepts is the "relaxation response" technique advocated by the Harvard Medical School cardiologist Dr. Herbert Benson. This approach is outlined in his books *The Relaxation Response, Beyond the Relaxation Response,* and *Your Maximum Mind.* In a capsule, Benson's approach may be described like this:

  1. Set aside about twenty minutes twice a day in a quiet place, where you're unlikely to be interrupted.

  2. Close your eyes and consciously relax all your major muscle groups.

*See, for example, Joel E. Dimsdale, "Anger and Blood Pressure," *Drug Therapy,* June 1989, pp. 105–109.

3. Concentrate on keeping your breathing regular.

4. Begin to repeat silently a soothing word or phrase, preferably one that is in harmony with your basic belief system. For example, a person from the Judeo-Christian tradition might pick a short Bible verse. The passage should be short enough so that the entire word or phrase can easily be repeated silently as you exhale.

5. When any outside thoughts threaten to interrupt your concentration—and you can be sure they will—don't fight them. Just gently turn away from the interruption and return to your breathing and your focus word.

This sequence should eventually evoke what Dr. Benson calls the "relaxation response," a measurable physical and emotional change, which often involves a lowering of heart rate and blood pressure. Benson emphasizes that regular breathing and a passive attitude are the keys to success with this relaxation technique.

Other relaxation techniques have also been found to be effective. Yoga, self-hypnosis, and biofeedback can produce mild reductions in blood pressure, especially in patients who tend to be anxious or tense and in young patients with mild hypertension.

Managing these risk factors can help prevent you from getting high blood pressure and can also help you control or reverse elevated readings you may now be experiencing. Of course, if your blood pressure does not respond to these non-pharmacological measures, further attention to your condition will be necessary.

Question 4: I've Got High Blood Pressure—So _____What Do I Do About It?_____

Despite making serious efforts to change their lives, many patients end up reciting a litany that goes like this: "I tried salt restriction. I stopped smoking and lost weight. I exercise moderately and use relaxation techniques. I have tried all the nonpharmacological methods to reduce the blood pressure. But my blood pressure is _still_ high. Now what do I do?" The answer is to get your physician to evaluate you for the anti-high-blood-pressure medications, and for all causes of hypertension.

The current generation of medicines that lower blood pressure is remarkable. Many new families of drugs have been introduced by pharmaceutical companies in response to the need for better antihypertension therapy. Ideally, the perfect medication would be 100 percent effective, safe, and convenient. It would produce few side effects, would require only a small dosage to be taken no more than once a day, and would be inexpensive.

Needless to say, such a perfect agent has not yet been found, and it possibly never will be. Still, the physician and patient now have medications that are more effective, with fewer side effects, than ever before. The prospects of correcting hypertension and preventing stroke have been greatly enhanced because of these drugs.

Many physicians will recommend that hypertension be treated through a series of clearly defined steps. As a result, the most recent approach to treatment is often called "step-care therapy." To understand better how this approach works, take a look at the diagram below, which has been produced by the Joint National Committee on Detection, Evaluation, and Treatment of High Blood Pressure.

Step-care therapy for hypertension (high blood pressure) involves the initiation of treatment with one of four classes of medicines. If the selected drug is ineffective or produces side effects, another drug can be substituted. If the drug is only

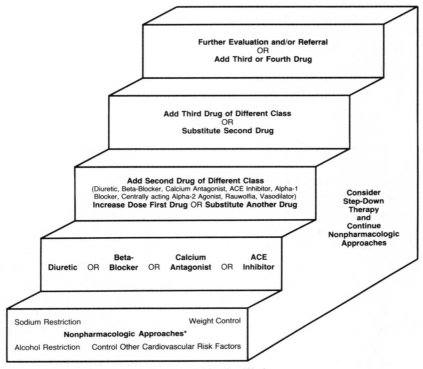

Further Evaluation and/or Referral
OR
Add Third or Fourth Drug

Add Third Drug of Different Class
OR
Substitute Second Drug

Add Second Drug of Different Class
(Diuretic, Beta-Blocker, Calcium Antagonist, ACE Inhibitor, Alpha-1 Blocker, Centrally acting Alpha-2 Agonist, Rauwolfia, Vasodilator)
Increase Dose First Drug OR Substitute Another Drug

Consider
Step-Down
Therapy
and
Continue
Nonpharmacologic
Approaches

		Beta-		Calcium		ACE
Diuretic	OR	Blocker	OR	Antagonist	OR	Inhibitor

Sodium Restriction   Weight Control
Nonpharmacologic Approaches*
Alcohol Restriction   Control Other Cardiovascular Risk Factors

*For some patients, nonpharmacologic therapy should be tried first. If goal blood pressure is not achieved, add pharmacologic therapy. Other patients may require pharmacologic therapy as initial treatment. In these instances, nonpharmacologic treatment may be a helpful adjunct.

Individualized Step-Care Therapy for Hypertension

partially effective, a second or third drug can be added in a systematic fashion.

As you can see from the diagram, which has been drawn in the shape of a staircase, there is a logical progression that treatment of hypertension should take. Assume that your physician will probably start you on the lowest step and then move up the staircase until he or she finds the combination of treatments that lowers your blood pressure measurements.

Step one: We have already dealt with the first step—which is labeled "Nonpharmacologic Approaches"—in our discussion of risk factors for high blood pressure. As pointed out, many people with mild or borderline hypertension (in the range of 140/90 to 159/94) will respond so well to this nondrug treatment that drugs aren't even necessary. Furthermore, even if medications are necessary, continuing with a nondrug approach will help keep the dosages of medication at a minimum.

Step two: If nondrug treatments fail to bring blood pressure into the normal range—and especially if measurements drift above the 159/94 level—some antihypertensive medications will probably be prescribed by your physician.

Note: You should assume that if *either* of these numbers, the systolic (upper) or diastolic (lower), drifts into the high blood pressure range, hypertension is present and some treatment is in order.

What drugs might your physician prescribe for this second step of treatment?

As you can see from the chart, four types of drugs are listed as possibilities for the second step of treatment—diuretics, beta-blockers, calcium antagonists (also known as calcium blockers or channel blockers), and ACE inhibitors. Because these are the most common antihypertensive drugs in use today, it is important if you have high blood pressure that you understand how each works, along with relevant side effects.

Diuretics. Commonly referred to as "water pills," a diuretic is an agent that increases the flow of urine. Most of these medications are lumped under the general category "thiazides." They are the most widely prescribed of all the antihypertensive drugs. But they have been losing ground in recent years to some of the newer medications. Diuretics reduce blood pressure primarily by causing the excretion of sodium from the body.

Common side effects of thiazide diuretics include a need to urinate frequently; a decline in sexual functioning in men; a loss of potassium, which can lead to irregular heart action; increase in blood sugar (glucose); elevation of uric acid in the blood; and an increase in blood fats, including cholesterol.

These drugs usually are *not* recommended for diabetics, for patients with gout, or for those with high blood fats, including cholesterol. If the electrocardiogram (ECG) shows irregular rhythms, it is also unlikely that thiazides will be used. Diuretics and calcium channel blockers have proven to be effective in black patients with hypertension.

Some drugs in the thiazide diuretic group include hydro-chlorthiazide (Esidrix), chlorthalidone (Hygroton), and most commonly used, chlorothiazide (Diuril).

Beta-blockers. There are two main ways that beta-block-ers, the second most prescribed medication after diuretics, act to reduce blood pressure. First, they slow the heart rate; they "block" adrenalinelike activity in the body. In addition, they re-duce the production of the enzyme renin in the kidneys. Renin helps increase the resistance of blood vessels to blood flow.

Side effects may include fatigue or lethargy, slow heart rates, insomnia, depression, and a reduction in HDL choles-terol, which has been linked to a higher incidence of coronary artery disease.

Those who may benefit most from beta-blockers include peo-ple with previous heart attacks; young patients with circula-tory problems; those with coronary artery disease; and those with significant anxiety, tremors, or irregular heartbeats. These drugs are *not* as effective in blacks as in whites. They are usually avoided in asthmatics and diabetics.

Some drugs in this group include propanalol (Inderal), aceb-utolol (Sectral), atenolol (Tenormin), and metoprolol (Lopres-sor).

Calcium blockers. These drugs, which are also called "channel blockers," "calcium channel blockers," and "calcium antagonists," lower blood pressure by cutting off the influx of calcium into the tiny channels in muscle cells in the wall of the artery. To contract, a muscle must have calcium; so without as much calcium, the vessels tend to remain more relaxed. As a result, there is less resistance to blood flow, and blood pressure is lowered. Not only do they lower blood pressure, these medi-cations may help prevent the progression of hardening of the arteries.

The side effects of calcium blockers may include headaches, swelling of the ankles, nausea, rashes or flushing, dizziness, and constipation. The side effects are not frequent. These drugs are usually prescribed for older people and are effective in black people. They are *not* typically recommended for people with irregular heartbeats or liver disease.

The drugs available in this group include verapamil (Calan), diltiazem (Cardizem), and nifedipine (Procardia). Newer ones are in the pipeline.

ACE inhibitors. The full name of these new drugs is "angiotensin *c*onverting *e*nzyme inhibitors" (hence the acronym ACE). They act primarily in the kidneys by inhibiting the action of a certain "converting" enzyme, which produces a substance known as angiotensin II. This angiotensin normally is a powerful constrictor of blood vessels. But by blocking the production of angiotensin, ACE inhibitors promote relaxation in the vessels. The result is a lower blood pressure.

Side effects of these drugs may include too-low blood pressure (hypotension), elevation of potassium in the blood, a loss of the sense of taste, impairment of kidney function, and a cough. The drugs are usually recommended for those with congestive heart failure and for younger people. The drugs may not be as effective in blacks, older people, and those with kidney problems.

Drugs in this group include lisinopril (Prinivil), captopril (Capoten), and enalapril (Vasotec). More are on the way.

Alpha blockers. These medications act by allowing the blood vessels to dilate, thereby reducing resistance to the flow of blood and hence a lowering of blood pressure.

An interesting side effect of this group of agents is a reduction in the size of the prostate gland in about 70 percent of males using these drugs. The reduction in the size of the prostate gland of aging males can indeed be a beneficial side effect, because it may remove the need for prostate surgery.

Drugs in this group include prazosin (Minipress) and terazosin (Hytrin).

Step three: The third step in the step-care therapy approach to high blood pressure must be taken if the nondrug treatments *and* the first application of drugs have failed to work. In general, this step involves one of three recommendations by your physician: (1) Increase the dosage of the first drug, (2) substitute another drug, or (3) *add* a second drug.

When substituting or adding a drug, any of the first four we have already discussed may be tried. For example, an ACE inhibitor may be substituted for a diuretic. Or a diuretic may be added to a beta-blocker.

In addition, other drugs, usually not appropriate for the first line of treatment, may now come into play. These include alpha-blockers (drugs that inhibit the action of receptors that cause tightness in the vessels), vasodilators (those that act directly to open up the blood vessels), and a miscellaneous variety of other medications.

Step four: If the therapy still hasn't succeeded in lowering blood pressure, a second drug may be substituted (if this step hasn't been taken already), or a third drug may be added.

Step five: A third or fourth drug may be added at this stage.

Finally, if drugs seem to be working after one of these steps has been completed, your physician may eventually consider "step-down therapy." This approach involves emphasizing nondrug treatments and cutting back gradually on dosages or an entire class of drugs. If the patient can maintain normal blood pressure with less medication, that will mean fewer side effects.

Many physicians prefer not to use the step-care approach to therapy. Some prefer to treat with one drug that they are familiar with—monotherapy. They will of course add to or modify the treatment based on the patient's response. Understanding all this is important so that you may better comprehend and cooperate with your physician's attempt to lower your blood pressure.

For the information of those patients who are actually taking medications, I have included a chart (Table 4). Common side effects, in nonmedical language as far as possible, are given.

If you have experienced a side effect or an untoward reaction to your medication, discuss it with your physician. He will evaluate your observation and determine whether another medication is indicated.

In some cases, a patient may do so well that medication may be discontinued entirely. But usually, patients with high blood pressure must plan on some sort of anti-high-blood-pressure monitoring throughout their lives. Remember the case of Ryan who went off his medication. He ended up with fairly consistent high blood pressure and worse.

Table 4. Common Oral Antihypertensive Drugs

Drug	Some Possible Side Effects
Thiazide and Related Diuretics	
Hydrochlorthiazide	Can elevate blood sugar and insulin resistance, lower serum potassium, lower libido; may increase serum uric acid; may increase fats in blood
Furosemide	Similar to hydrochlorthiazide
Spironolactone	Breast enlargement and decreased libido in men; menstrual irregularity; muscle weakness; nausea and vomiting
Triamterene	Nausea, high potassium in blood, with muscle weakness and numbness
Amiloride	Nausea, high potassium in blood, with muscle weakness and numbness
Beta-Blockers	
Propranolol	Asthma, cold hands and feet, vivid dreams, masking of insulin reactions, fatigue, decreased libido
Metoprolol	Same as propranolol, but less bronchial constriction and less masking of insulin reactions
Nadolol	Similar to propanolol
Atenolol	Same as metoprolol
Timolol	Same as propanolol
Pindolol	Same as propanolol, but less slowing of the heart
Acebutolol	Same as metoprolol and pindolol
Betaxolol	Same as metoprolol and pindolol
Labetalol	Same as propanolol, but also nausea, indigestion; dizziness may occur initially
Drugs Acting as Brain Centers	
Methyldopa	Sleepiness, fever, tiredness, hepatitis, anemia, dry mouth

Drug	Some Possible Side Effects
Clonidine (available in skin patches)	Sedation, dry mouth, dizziness, weakness, lower libido; can decrease withdrawal symptoms from nicotine
Guanabenz	Same as clonidine
Guanfacine	Same as clonidine

Alpha-Blockers

Prazosin	Dizziness or fainting when assuming upright position
Terazosin	Same as prazosin

Vasodilators

Hydralazine	Rapid and sometimes irregular heartbeats, nausea, headache, dizziness; prolonged use may cause lupus reaction—fever, joint pains
Minoxidil	Increase in hair on face, dizziness, headache, swelling of feet

ACE Inhibitors

Captopril	Cough, increased serum potassium, skin rash, low white blood count, taste changes, dizziness, weakness
Enalapril	Same as captopril
Lisinopril	Same as captopril

Calcium Channel Blockers

Nifedipine	Rapid heart action, dizziness, nausea, headache, swelling of feet, redness of face and neck
Diltiazem	Constipation, swelling of feet, headache, nausea, tiredness
Verapamil	Constipation, slowing of heart, headache, swelling of feet
Nicardipine	Same as nifedipine

The most important point to remember as we leave the subject is this: High blood pressure is a major, if not *the* major, risk factor for stroke. So it is essential to do whatever you can to prevent the onset of high blood pressure or to reduce it if you have it. Such action may very well save your life.

Chapter Six

The Ultimate Attack Strategy for Artery Disease

Narrowed and blocked arteries that feed blood to the brain are the most common cause of stroke. The deadly drama that can threaten health and life often unfolds like this: Fatty particles, along with their protein encasings, become embedded in the artery walls, and over the years, they build up in an accumulation known as plaque. Slowly and insidiously, the plaque reduces the blood flow to the brain.

The narrowed vessel struggles to provide the brain with oxygen and nutrients. This internal lifeline is absolutely necessary to maintain mental and nervous functions at acceptable levels. If the channel in the narrowed vessel is too small to allow passage, the clotted material will lodge in the opening and shut off the blood flow.

The result will be a stroke. With a stroke, the part of the brain normally fed by a clogged artery fails to receive its required nourishment and oxygen, and the affected tissue begins to die. This type of stroke is called a "cerebral thrombosis" or "cerebral infarction." Consider the illustrations below, depicting the gradual narrowing of an artery.

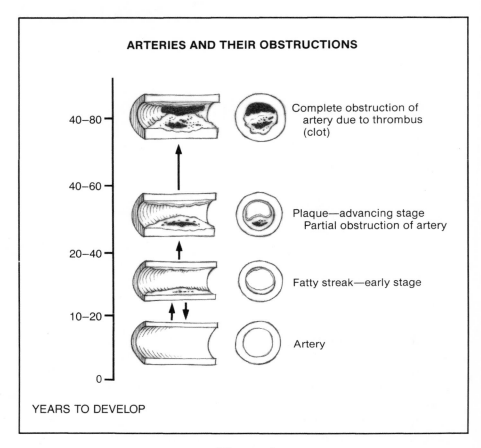

ARTERIES AND THEIR OBSTRUCTIONS

Complete obstruction of
artery due to thrombus
(clot)

Plaque—advancing stage
Partial obstruction of artery

Fatty streak—early stage

Artery

YEARS TO DEVELOP

Figure 4
The Buildup of Plaque in an Artery

What Causes Narrowing
_____of the Arteries?_____

There are several possible sources of the artery disease that
may result in stroke. Here are a few of the factors that should
be considered by all who are concerned about the prevention
of a dreaded stroke.

Source 1: Natural blood fat production. The liver produces an estimated 70–80 percent of cholesterol and other fatty molecules that circulate through the bloodstream. Yet the bodies of some people naturally produce more blood fats, including cholesterol, than those of other people. Those who tend to put out more blood fats will often have excessively high cholesterol levels—and therein lies a major danger of stroke and heart disease.

Cholesterol in a capsule. Pure cholesterol is a waxy substance. It is absorbed from our diet by the intestine. A nondietary amount that circulates in our blood is formed in many cells of the body, but especially in the liver, where it is used to make bile salts and bile acids. This is called "endogenous cholesterol." (That which comes in from the diet is known as "exogenous cholesterol.")

About 80 percent of the total cholesterol, from all sources, is then converted to other uses. Small quantities of cholesterol are used by the adrenal gland, ovaries, and testes to manufacture hormones, the ovaries and testes. A larger amount of cholesterol is in our skin. It helps make the skin resistant to substances that might be injurious and helps control the evaporation of water from the skin.

Cholesterol is packaged in the bloodstream in a combination of protein and fat called lipoproteins. The lipoproteins can disperse freely in the bloodstream, whereas cholesterol itself cannot. There are two important lipoproteins. The "bad" one is known as low-density lipoprotein (LDL). The other, "good" one is high-density lipoprotein (HDL).

The concentration of LDL is regulated by LDL *receptors,* which develop as a result of commonly inherited genes. If these receptor cells are not inherited, a high level of cholesterol and LDL in the blood will result. Also, a high-fat, high-cholesterol diet may overwhelm the LDL receptors and lead to high cholesterol and LDL in the blood. In addition, such a diet signals the body to manufacture fewer LDL receptors.

You might think of the LDL receptors as a sponge that soaks up excess cholesterol on its way to disposal by the body. If not enough receptors are present, or if the amount of cholesterol presented to the receptors by a cholesterol-rich diet is overwhelming, the sponge becomes saturated and ineffective. Hence serum cholesterol will rise in the blood and be deposited in the arteries.

The function of the "good" HDL cholesterol seems to be to "mop up" extra LDL cholesterol that has been missed by the receptors. HDLs thus help eliminate excess "bad" LDLs from the bloodstream. The more HDLs you have in relation to your LDLs, the better.

The average total cholesterol level for American adults now hovers around 215 to 225 mg/dl, a range that is down significantly from the 235-plus reading of a few years ago. Education of the public about the dangers of high cholesterol has certainly had an important impact, but we still have a long way to go. Recent studies have shown that total cholesterol should be no more than 200 mg/dl in adults above the age of twenty. In fact, the risk of cardiovascular disease rises by 2 percent for every 1 mg/dl that a person's cholesterol rises above the 200 level. Some so-called primitive societies where hardening of the arteries is virtually nonexistent have cholesterol levels between 130 and 160 mg/dl.

Are those with a naturally higher production of cholesterol destined almost inevitably for a stroke or other vessel disease problem? By no means! A bit later, we will review a number of preventive approaches that may be taken, including changing diet and life-style and the use of medically supervised medications. But first, let's take a look at the second source of plaque buildup—the diet.

Source 2: A high-fat, high-cholesterol diet. Remember this key point: Your body makes enough cholesterol so that you do not need additional cholesterol from your diet. Yet about 20–30 percent of cholesterol in the bloodstream comes from dietary sources.

Another key point: When you are evaluating your diet, it's important to distinguish between foods high in fats and foods high in cholesterol. Also, it is necessary to distinguish between different types of fats because not all fats have the same impact on blood cholesterol. As you'll see, there are three types of fats in your diet: (1) Saturated fats, which tend to be solid at room temperature, are bad for you because they tend to raise cholesterol levels. (2) Monounsaturated fats, such as olive oil, may actually lower cholesterol. (3) Polyunsaturated fats, such as corn oil, may also help lower cholesterol.

To understand these points, let's consider the diet of Mary T., who assiduously avoided as much cholesterol as possible in planning her menus. Her objective: to lower her blood cholesterol level, which had been measured at 238 in her most recent blood test. She managed to keep her cholesterol intake in the range of about 150 milligrams per day by avoiding eggs and by buying supermarket foods that were clearly labeled "no cholesterol," or "cholesterol-free." By this dietary plan, she reduced her intake of cholesterol from an average of about 450 milligrams per day to 150. So she was understandably upset when she went in for her next blood test and discovered that the reading had actually gone *up,* to 265 mg/dl!

What had gone wrong? The problem was that in reducing her cholesterol intake, Mary had increased her consumption of saturated fats. (Saturated fats are found in meats, dairy products, and tropical oils.) Through a biochemical process in the body, saturated fats, even in foods that contain no cholesterol, will often trigger dramatic rises of cholesterol in the blood.

That's what happened to Mary. She had increased her consumption of potato chips and other foods that were high in saturated fats. Also, she had included more foods containing palm oil and coconut oil, which though vegetable in origin are perhaps the *worst* because they raise blood cholesterol levels. She thought that because a food was labeled "no cholesterol," it had to be okay.

After some nutritional counseling, Mary designed a diet that was much lower in cholesterol *and* in fats—especially saturated fats. Furthermore, she cut out egg yolks and fried food, and switched to fat-free dairy products. She used "no oil" salad dressings. This approach was consistent with recent studies showing that monounsaturated fats (such as those in canola and olive oil) may actually lower blood cholesterol. Polyunsaturated fats (for example, corn, walnut, safflower, and soybean oil) may also help lower cholesterol levels. As a result of these changes in her diet, Mary's next blood test showed that her total cholesterol had dropped to a respectable 190 mg/dl.

Table 5. Dietary Sources of Saturated Fats and Low-Fat Substitutes

Category	Item	Saturated Fat (g)	Cholesterol (mg)
Meats			
	Ground beef patty cooked, regular, 4 oz	9.2	102
	Turkey, light, roasted skinless, 4 oz	1.2	78
Eggs			
	Egg yolk, 1	1.7	215
	Commercial egg substitute	0	0
Dairy			
Cheese	American cheese, 1 oz	6	30
	Substitute cheese	1	0
Milk	Milk, whole, 1 cup	5.1	33
	Milk, skim, 1 cup	0.6	5
Cream	Ice cream, 1 cup	9	60
	Nonfat yogurt, 1 cup	0.3	Trace
Invisible fats (as in baked goods, snacks)			
	Doughnut, 1 piece	5	20
	French fries, 1 order	7	15
	Fruits	0	0
Cooking/table fats			
	Butter, 1 T	7	30
	Soft diet margarine, 1 T	1	0
	Hard margarine (stick), 1 T	2.1	0
	Coconut oil, 1 T	11.8	0
	Corn oil, 1 T	1.7	0
Snacks			
	Peanuts, dry-roasted, ¼ cup	3.1	0
	Popcorn, salted, buttered, 3 cups	2.7	12
	Popcorn, 3 cups	Trace	0
	Chocolate chip cookies, 2	1.3	8

Values are approximate and taken from standard food tables.

Table 5 shows how some representative foods can affect your intake of cholesterol *and* saturated fats. By reviewing this table, you can tell at a glance what is best to eat. Note that saturated fats raise your cholesterol more than anything in your diet. And remember, they are found in animal sources and whole milk products. Some examples include butter and cheese, beef, pork, poultry skin, coconut oil, and palm oil. Also, you should be alert to the word "hydrogenated" on your food labels. Hydrogenation is a process that converts liquid oils to a more solid form—and that results in more saturation. So try to use foods that contain less saturated fat than polyunsaturated fat.

Here are a few more food tips that will help you lower your blood cholesterol:

* Polyunsaturated oils are also found in fish. Cold water fish such as mackerel, salmon, and herring have abundant fat. Warm water fish such as red snapper and flounder are relatively low in total fat. But both groups of fish are low in saturated fat.

* Foods rich in cholesterol are of animal origin. Egg yolk, organ meats, and shrimp are relatively high in cholesterol.

* Fiber and complex carbohydrates are excellent substitutes for foods high in saturated fatty acids and cholesterol. Fiber is the material from plant walls that does not undergo digestion.

    Pasta (not pizza), breads, cereals, peas, beans, fruits, and vegetables are good sources. Higher-fiber diets containing barley, oat bran, beans, vegetables, and fruits not only lower total serum cholesterol but may raise levels of the "good" HDL cholesterol.

Source 3: Damage to the blood vessels during aging.

As mentioned in the preceding chapter on hypertension, a blood pressure reading that stays too high over a period of time can do damage to the inner walls of the blood vessels. The chips, tears, and roughening that occur through this process probably make the vessels more vulnerable to the accumulation of fatty material from the blood. The end result is the buildup of plaque that obstructs a vessel.

Apart from high blood pressure, however, the mere process of aging and plaque formation do damage to the vessels by a process that has come to be known as "hardening of the arteries." In fact, in common parlance, this term has come to be synonymous with atherosclerosis or arteriosclerosis.

Let's further define the terms. *Atherosclerosis* is a disease of the arteries in which fatty plaques develop in the inside of the arteries. Along with plaque on the inside, there is a great amount of connective tissue in the wall of the artery, and as the body ages, the connective tissue loses elasticity so that the arteries become relatively rigid and unyielding. This process is called *sclerosis*. Still later, calcium salts are deposited, leading to bony, hard arteries that are like rigid tubes. These stages are referred to as hardening of the arteries. The entire process is thus called *arteriosclerosis*.

What happens during this hardening process? One of the features of the aging process is the loss of many elastic fibers throughout the body. As an example, the skin sags because of an ongoing rupture of fibers that support the skin. Therefore, as we age, we wrinkle more. Similarly, there is a loss of elasticity in the vascular system. The result of the process is a loss of elasticity in the vessels and degeneration of the walls of the arteries, so that they are more likely to become damaged as we age.

What Should Be ___Your Cholesterol Targets?___

When you have a blood test, there are four cholesterol figures that are of concern to you: (1) total cholesterol; (2) "bad" cholesterol, also known as low-density lipoprotein (LDL) cholesterol; (3) "good cholesterol," also known as high-density lipoprotein (HDL) cholesterol; (4) the ratio of total cholesterol to HDL cholesterol; and (5) the total fats in the blood—the triglycerides.

When tests are performed to determine the amount of fats

in the blood, the tests are often referred to as a "lipid profile." The total cholesterol includes the LDL cholesterol (the bad kind), plus the HDL cholesterol (the good), plus about 20 percent of the total triglycerides (other fats) in the blood.

The lipid profile is often reported in terms of total cholesterol, the LDL (though some labs don't automatically give you this figure), HDL, and serum triglycerides. Usually, you have to figure out your total cholesterol to HDL cholesterol ratio. (The calculation: Divide total cholesterol by your HDL cholesterol. So if your total cholesterol is 200 and your HDLs are 50, your ratio is 4.0.)

In general, you can simplify the meaning of these figures if you keep these guidelines in mind: Your total cholesterol should be low (less than 200); your LDL should be as low as possible (below 130—see the chart later in this chapter); your HDL should be high (above 45–50); and your triglycerides should be low (below about 120).

Framingham researchers have reported that those between the ages of forty-nine and eighty-two who tend to have high HDLs also have a lower risk of cardiovascular disease. Other studies show that individuals in their eighties and nineties have low levels of LDL and high levels of HDL.

The National Cholesterol Education Program (NCEP) guidelines suggest that the total cholesterol level for adults above twenty years of age should be less than 200 mg/dl. On the other hand, if the total cholesterol is high, an elevated HDL level might be protective.

Note: A serum cholesterol level of 200 is not a magic number. It is just a statistical figure that attempts risk prediction. That is, a serum cholesterol reading under 200 is less likely to be associated with heart attacks and strokes.

There has been recent controversy over whether low cholesterol in the blood is causally related to suicides, aggressive behavior, and other disorders. The supporters of such theories, which are based on inadequate studies, may jeopardize the lives of many people. Those who seek an excuse to pooh-pooh a cutback in cholesterol and fatty foods will be tempted to ignore sound anthropological, epidemiological, animal, and human data and eat their way into oblivion.

Note: Diet is to heart disease what blood pressure is to

stroke. Cholesterol values are more closely correlated to heart attacks, whereas high blood pressure parallels stroke incidence more closely. The combination of high cholesterol and high blood pressure predisposes one to both illnesses—the younger person to heart disease, the older to stroke.

Total cholesterol. As already indicated, the desired total cholesterol target for most adults is below 200 mg/dl. Those with less than 200 mg/dl—and normal to high HDLs—don't need to be concerned about their total cholesterol.

In 1985, the National Heart, Lung, and Blood Institute initiated the National Cholesterol Education Program to encourage everyone to know their cholesterol level and if elevated, try to do something about it.

Those with a measurement of total cholesterol in the borderline 200–239 range should take dietary steps to lower their readings. They should also pay close attention to the subcomponents of their cholesterol, including the LDL and HDL levels. As previously noted, this range becomes even more ominous if the patient has other risk factors for stroke, such as high blood pressure.

Finally, people with a total cholesterol reading of 240 or higher should submit to close medical supervision to lower this figure. Elevated cholesterol may be caused by low thyroid activity (hypothyroidism) and kidney disease (nephrosis). If dietary or life-style changes don't work, drug treatments will be required.

The specter of LDL cholesterol. Most experts believe that it is even more important to focus on total *LDL* cholesterol (the "bad" component) than on total cholesterol. The reason: Total cholesterol is made up of several components, some of which (especially HDL) are good for you. So identifying the level of the bad LDLs will help to target more precisely what your real problem is—and what must be done about it. As we'll see shortly, it is the LDL cholesterol that tends to be most responsive to a low-fat, low-cholesterol diet.

The objective should be to bring your LDL cholesterol below 130 mg/dl. One way to do that is through the dietary changes that have already been discussed in this chapter. (See also "Tactic 1: Life-style Change," below.)

"Good" cholesterol. Your third cholesterol target—after total cholesterol and LDL cholesterol—concerns the "good" cholesterol, or high-density lipoprotein (HDL) cholesterol. In general, the higher your HDL level, the better, because HDL cholesterol is believed to be protective against clogging of the arteries (atherosclerosis). Scientists aren't quite sure how this works: Some believe that HDLs act as a kind of "garbage removal" system to get rid of excess LDL cholesterol. They say that a ten-milligram elevation of HDL can result in a 50-percent reduction in risk.

Whatever the mechanism, it is a fact that families with markedly elevated HDL have less cardiovascular disease. In one study, a woman was found to have an HDL level of 225 (five times the average) and a serum cholesterol of 100. There is a history of longevity and no cardiovascular disease on both sides of her family. Because of these findings, this woman being studied was considered by some observers to have a kind of "Methuselah gene," which virtually ensures long life by preventing atherosclerosis. Time will tell.

What are the desirable HDL levels? The average for men is about 45 mg/dl, while the average for women is about 55 mg/dl. As women grow older and move through menopause, their level of HDL tends to decline, perhaps because of the loss of their ability to produce estrogen. High levels of estrogen have been associated with higher levels of HDL cholesterol. So if you are a man and your HDL measurement is below 45, you should try to bring it up. Likewise, women with HDL levels below 55 should try to raise the reading.

How can you raise your HDL cholesterol? Diet doesn't seem to work as effectively as it does in lowering LDL cholesterol. Still, some other changes in life-style can be made to raise HDL levels. For example, weight reduction occasionally results in elevation of HDL levels, and increasing the amount of time spent in aerobic exercise will tend to raise HDL levels. Also, cigarette smoking operates to decrease the HDL levels, so breaking the habit may raise the HDL. A very modest amount of alcohol may be of help too in raising the HDL.

Now, here is a summary of the HDL-raising possibilities that don't involve medications:

* Regular endurance (aerobic) exercise, such as jogging, swimming, cycling, or vigorous walking for at least twenty minutes per day, three to four days per week.

* Stopping smoking immediately.

* Loss of excess weight.

* Light alcohol consumption (up to one ounce per day). Obviously, this approach is *not* recommended for those with an alcohol problem.

* Eating fish that contains fatty acids known as "omega-3 fatty acids." (Some evidence suggests that eating fish such as salmon, mackerel, tuna, and sardines may help raise HDL levels.)

The ratio. Finally, the ratio of total cholesterol to HDL cholesterol is a mathematical way to express biological findings. The basic rule for the ratio is the lower the better. As for specific numbers, a ratio of 5.0 or below for men is in the acceptable range. The desirable range for women is 4.5 or below. Here are some examples that demonstrate how the ratio works.

* Tom R. had a total cholesterol reading of 230 and HDL cholesterol of 40. To determine his ratio we would divide 230 by 40. That results in a ratio of 5.75, too high to qualify for the good or safe range. Tom will either have to lower his total cholesterol (as through a low-fat, low-cholesterol diet) or raise his HDL cholesterol (as described above), or do both.

* Rhonda B. learned that her total cholesterol was 195, and her HDL cholesterol was 62. This meant that her ratio was a *very* healthy 3.15. Since she has no other risk factors, her risk of cardiovascular disease including stroke is considered to be low.

How to Conquer Your
____Vessel-Clogging Problems____

Now, we come to the essence of the "Ultimate Attack Strategy" to combat the artery disease that may lead to heart attack and stroke. There are two main tactics in this strategy: life-style change, and medications.

Tactic 1: Life-style Change

We have already explored some ways that your life-style can be altered so as to help prevent a stroke through clogging of the arteries. At this point, let me expand further upon those approaches and also add a few new ones.

Achieve a low-fat diet. This life-style change can be accomplished by elimination and addition. Some illustrations:

Eliminate whole milk products, but add skim milk products. Also, choose 1-percent-fat cottage cheese instead of 2- or 4-percent; nonfat yogurt; nonfat ice creams; and nonfat frozen yogurts. Eliminate foods containing egg yolks. Substitute those made with the whites of eggs. Cakes, waffles, pancakes, and mayonnaise are now available without egg yolk and the attendant cholesterol.

The accompanying table can give you an idea of the content of cholesterol and fat of common foods. Our objective should be to reduce the cholesterol intake as well as the intake of saturated fat in our diet. As previously mentioned, the absence of cholesterol in a food does not necessarily confer blessings on that food. For example, there is no cholesterol in coconut oil but there is plenty of "bad" saturated fat. Your cholesterol intake should be less than 300 grams per day. Your saturated fat intake should be less than 10 percent of your daily caloric need.

Eliminate butter and fried foods. Add jelly or jam on bread. Eliminate high-saturated-fat meats (veal, lamb, pork) and organ meats (brains, kidneys, liver). Add protein-rich, fat-poor fish.

To help you select some good fish dishes for your eating program, I have included Table 6 of common fish, with fat content, cholesterol content, and omega-3 fatty acids indicated. These fish oils came into prominence because of studies that demonstrated less deaths from heart disease in Greenland Eskimos compared with Danes.

Table 6. Common Fish Dishes with Fat Contents

Food*	Fat (g)	Cholesterol (mg)	Omega-3 Fatty Acids (g)
Catfish	3.1	55	0.3
Clams	1.5	40	0.1
Cod	0.7	40	0.2
Crab (Dungeness)	1.3	59	0.3
Crab (imitation)	0.1	50	0.2
Flounder	1.4	50	0.2
Haddock	0.5	60	0.2
Halibut	1.2	50	0.4
Lobster	1.7	85	0.2
Monkfish	1.0	35	NA
Mussels	1.6	25	0.5
Ocean perch	1.5	60	0.2
Orange roughy	0.3	58	0.1
Oysters	1.2	50	0.6
Rockfish (snapper)	1.8	40	0.5
Sablefish (black cod)	5.7	65	1.5
Salmon	7.0	65	1.1
Scallops	0.2	50	0.2
Shark (thrasher)	4.5	51	0.8
Shrimp	0.8	158	0.3
Sole	0.5	45	0.1
Squid	0.9	230	0.4
Swordfish	4.4	50	0.2
Trout (rainbow)	11.4	50	0.5
Tuna (albacore)	3.0	25	1.3

NOTE: Adapted with permission from Harsila, J., and Hansen, E., *Seafood: A Collection of Heart-Healthy Recipes*, 1985; and *Light-Hearted Seafood*, 1989. Richmond Beach, Washington, National Seafood Educators.
*3.5 oz of the raw, edible portion.

NOTE: Reprinted, by permission, from *The Physician and Sportsmedicine*, Vol. 18, No. 4 (April 1990), p. 20.

The increased use of fish to twice a week or more is recommended because of its low-fat content and the presence of omega-3 fatty acids.

Go for high-fiber foods. This dietary point is an important companion to the low-fat principle because the more fiber you take in, the fewer high-fat foods you tend to eat. Popular synonyms for fiber, by the way, are the terms *roughage* and *bulk*.

Your goal should be to increase your intake of dietary fiber to greater than twenty-five grams per day. The use of wheat and cereal bran is one of the primary methods of increasing dietary fiber. This can be accomplished by eating one-quarter to one-half cups of bran daily.

Additionally, you should increase your consumption of whole grain products. Eating fruits and vegetables, especially those with edible skins, contributes to the goal of increasing the fiber content of your diet. Table 7 can be used as a guide to your selection of fiber-containing food.

There are numerous studies that suggest that certain types of fibers—known as soluble fibers—can have an independent impact in lowering cholesterol levels in the blood. Specifically, it has been suggested that oats and oat bran can lower cholesterol levels. Other foods containing significant amounts of soluble fiber include dried beans and citrus fruits.

To be effective, these products must be consumed in considerable quantity. For example, a study at Northwestern University Medical School showed that if the average person consumes 35 grams of oat bran or oatmeal a day, he can lower his cholesterol by about 3 percent. How much actual food must you eat to take in 35 grams? One ounce of pure oat bran cereal (two thirds of a cup, cooked) or one ounce of oatmeal (two thirds of a cup, cooked) weighs 28 grams. So, as you can see, you'll need a little more than an ounce to reach the 35-gram level.

If you want to lower your cholesterol even further, you can consume even *more* soluble fiber. For example, reductions in cholesterol averaging about 10 percent have occurred in those eating 100 grams (a little more than 3 ounces) per day of oat bran, either in the form of muffins or cereal.

Table 7. Dietary Fiber Content of Selected Foods

	Grams per Serving			
	0.5 or less	0.5–1.0	1.1–2.0	2.1–3.0	3.0 or greater‡

Fruit*†

0.5 or less	0.5–1.0	1.1–2.0	2.1–3.0	3.0 or greater‡
Banana	Apricots,	Blueberries	Blackberries	Elderberries (5)
Cherries	Apple (raw, dried)	Coconut (fresh)	Boysenberries	Guava (5)
Coconumt (shred)	Applesauce	Currants (raw)	Pears (dried)	Raspberries
Currants (dried)	Cantaloupe	Gooseberries		
Dates	Cranberries (raw)	Papaya		
Fruit juice	Grapefruit	Pear		
Plums (cooked)	Grapes	Strawberries		
Pomegranate	Kiwifruit			
Prunes	Mango			
Raisins	Nectarine			
Watermelon	Orange			
Rhubarb (raw)	Peach			
	Pineapple			
	Plums (raw)			
	Rhubarb (cooked)			
	Tangerine			

Vegetables*†

0.5 or less	0.5–1.0	1.1–2.0	2.1–3.0	3.0 or greater‡
Bamboo shoots	Asparagus	Artichoke		
Bean sprouts	Beans (string)	Broccoli (cooked)		
Cabbage	Carrots	Brussels sprouts		
Celery	Beets	Pumpkin		
Endive	Broccoli (raw)	Sauerkraut		
Mushrooms	Cauliflower	Chicory (raw)		
Onions	Cucumber			
Parsley	Eggplant			
Radishes	Greens (cooked)			
Summer squash	Beet			
Vegetable juice	Collard			

Water chestnuts
Watercress
Dandelion
Kale
Mustard
Spinach
Swiss chard
Turnip
Green pepper
Kohlrabi
Okra
Rutabaga
Soybean sprouts
Spinach (raw)
Tomato
Turnips

Starches[*][†][‡]

Cornflakes	Granola	Black-eyed peas	40% Branflakes	All-Bran (13)
Corn grits	Oatmeal (cooked)	Brown bread	Bulgur	Bran Buds (12)
Cream of wheat, rice, and corn	Spaghetti and macaroni from whole wheat flour	Brown rice	Parsnips	100% Bran (9)
Farina	White bread	Cheerios	Raisin Bran	Bran muffin (3.5)
Graham crackers	White flour	Grape-Nuts	Ry-Krisp	Dried kidney beans (5)
Maltomeal	White rice	Green peas	Shredded Wheat	Dried navy beans (5)
Potato chips	White roll or bun	Popcorn	Wheat germ	Dried peas (5)
Potatoes		Ralston (cooked cereal)		Lentils (3.1)
Puffed cereals		Sesame seed kernels		Wheat bran (4)
Rice Krispies		Soybeans		
Saltines		Split peas		
Spaghetti		Total		
		Wheat Chex		

*Based on the content of one diabetic exchange for each item listed.
†Includes all forms (raw, dried, cooked) for fruits and vegetables except where noted.
‡Actual dietary fiber content listed in parentheses.
NOTE: Reprinted, by permission, from *Mayo Clinic Diet Manual*, "Nutritional Management of Diseases and Disorders," pp. 143–44.

Caution: Eating a high-fiber diet before your gastrointestinal system is used to these foods may cause gas, diarrhea, or other intestinal problems. So it is best to embark on a high-fiber diet *gradually*.

Also, you should ascertain what other food products, such as fats, are contained in the high-fiber dishes. For example, a very high-fiber oat bran muffin may be prepared with high-fat, high-cholesterol ingredients such as butter and eggs. The result may be that even though you increase your intake of soluble fiber, you *also* increase your consumption of calories, fat, and cholesterol. So learn how your food is prepared!

Try some "cutting-edge" foods and supplements. Another easy way to change your life-style for the better—and also minimize your risk of having an artery-blocking stroke— is to try the supplement route. The final scientific word isn't in yet on how supplements and other special foods may be of benefit in preventing stroke. But preliminary reports indicate that certain supplements, when taken in reasonable quantities, apparently can't do you any harm—and may actually do some good.

For example, antioxidants may be helpful. These substances have played important roles as food preservatives and in a variety of other uses. Probucol, a medication for lowering cholesterol, has actually been used to prevent oxidation in auto tires! The tires are hardier and last longer. But more important for our purposes, preventing the oxidation of LDLs is another way, independent of diet, for lowering serum cholesterol and thus retarding the atherosclerotic process. Unfortunately, food processing often destroys natural antioxidants. Also, many people consume little vitamin E, vitamin C, or betacarotene (a precursor of vitamin A). Eating habits should be cultivated to take in more of these vitamins through cereals, vitamin-E-rich oils, vegetables, and fruits.

Low-density lipoproteins, the major "bad" component of cholesterol, are subject to modification in the body through oxidation. This modified version, called "oxidized LDL," activates the atherosclerotic process. Specifically, oxidized LDL becomes "bound" to scavenger receptors. These cells promote atherosclerosis in animals and humans. On the other hand, blocking the oxidation of LDL by taking the antioxidants may slow down the atherosclerotic process. This blocking action has been shown to occur in experimental animals and is also believed to happen in humans.

Vitamin E, vitamin C, and betacarotene are potent antioxidants. Here are a few suggestions for making these "cutting edge" substances a part of your Ultimate Attack Strategy on stroke:

Become an ACE user. An easy way to remember how to attack the artery-clogging type of stroke through supplements is this: Make sure that your diet contains an "ACE"—vitamins A, C, and E—on a daily basis. (This ACE is not to be confused with the ACE inhibitors used in the treatment of high blood pressure.)

Apart from its beneficial effects on our eyes and skin, the plant precursors of vitamin A, the carotenoids (including betacarotene), are believed to help neutralize the oxidation of "bad" LDL cholesterol. Also, vitamin A precursors have been found to decrease the incidence of cancers of the mouth, throat, larynx (voice box), and lung. So consider taking 25,000 IUs (international units) daily.

Vitamin C also has a cancer-fighting quality, but our main interest in this discussion is in its potential for reducing serum cholesterol as antioxidants. Additionally, vitamin C is important in giving our connective and supporting tissues stability and strength. How much should you take? Consider taking 500 milligrams twice a day. Dr. Linus Pauling recommends much more.

The National Center for Health Statistics has found that a relatively high vitamin C intake leads to a reduction in deaths due to cardiovascular diseases and cancer, possibly through the mechanism of its antioxidant properties.

Alpha tocopherol is the most active of the seven forms of vitamin E and is widely distributed in green plants. Rich sources of vitamin E include whole wheat products and wheat germ. Because vitamin E is a potent antioxidant that may help slow down the atherosclerotic process, consider taking 400 IUs daily.

Vitamin B_6 is another possibility. It comes in three forms, pyridoxine, pyridoxamine, and pyridoxal. Uncooked grains and legumes contain significant amounts. It has long been known that monkeys fed a diet deficient in B_6 develop atherosclerosis. Human studies are currently in progress on this issue. Note: Refrigeration, canning, and refining destroy vitamin B_6. Twenty-five mg of vitamin B_6 daily may be helpful.

Caution: Check with your physician before taking any supplement. Even though the general population may be safe taking such supplements, your personal medical history will be reviewed by your physician. It would be best if your diet provided you with sufficient vitamins, minerals, and nutrients since supplements are so costly.

Finally, you might increase your consumption of garlic. Some preliminary studies support anecdotal folklore that suggests that garlic can help prevent clots in the bloodstream. Controlled studies are needed to determine whether garlic lowers blood pressure and has other beneficial effects.

Increase your participation in aerobic exercise. The final kind of life-style change that can reduce your risk for an artery-blocking type of stroke is exercise.

As I have mentioned above (see the discussion of the subcomponents of cholesterol), "good" HDL cholesterol is often positively affected by endurance exercise, such as jogging, cycling, and vigorous walking. To obtain significant benefits, however, don't overdo it.

A study conducted by the Institute for Aerobics Research in Dallas and published in the *Journal of the American Medical Association* in 1989 shows that walking only about thirty minutes a day, three days a week, can have major benefits in reducing the rate of deaths resulting from vascular problems, as well as from other diseases. One of the main reasons for the benefits to those at risk from strokes or heart attacks seems to be that this type of exercise helps raise the level of HDL cholesterol, which as you now know has been linked to protection against vascular diseases. The concept that you can "run off" or "burn off" your cholesterol is dangerous and wrong.

Making these and related life-style changes has helped many people significantly reduce their risk of stroke. But sometimes, more is needed—and that is where our second major tactic comes in. In a great number of cases, it is necessary for the patient's physician to intervene and prescribe drugs to help battle and conquer the cholesterol and atherosclerosis challenge.

Tactic 2: Prescription Drugs

When should medication be considered to lower blood cholesterol levels? In general, if the levels of "bad" LDL cholesterol are above 160 milligrams per deciliter and attempts to make life-style changes don't work, medications may be appropriate. If total cholesterol is above 240 mg/dl, medication may be prescribed—though the LDL level and the total cholesterol to HDL cholesterol ratio will also be considered. If the HDL levels are quite high and the LDL cholesterol relatively low, there is less concern about a somewhat high total cholesterol level. The cholesterol/HDL ratio will be reflective.

What types of medication are likely to be selected? The main objective is to find a drug or combination of drugs that (1) lowers LDL cholesterol; (2) raises or at least maintains original levels of HDL cholesterol; and (3) produces minimal side effects. Some of the main categories—which are indicated in Table 8—include the following:

Niacin. This over-the-counter preparation, also known as nicotinic acid or vitamin B_3, can be obtained without a prescription. It often lowers LDL cholesterol while maintaining levels of HDL cholesterol or even raising them. Typically, niacin must be taken in relatively large doses, with a one- to two-gram minimum, to achieve beneficial effects.

Warning: Although niacin can be obtained without a doctor's prescription, it should *never* be taken without a doctor's recommendation and supervision. The problem is that some people have suffered severe liver damage from this drug. There may be other side effects, such as flushing, rashes, or possibly irregular heartbeats. The side effects of niacin may be so disturbing as to prevent its effective use in lowering cholesterol.

Resins. These prescription drugs bind the bile acids produced by the liver and help the excretion of cholesterol from

Table 8. Characteristics of the Major Medications That Lower or Adjust Cholesterol and Other Fats in the Blood

Drug	Possible side effects	Dosage
Cholestyramine (Questran)	Constipation, bloating	Starting 4 g/d; range 12–24 g/d
Colestipol HCl (Colestid)	Constipation, bloating	Starting 5 g/d; range 15–30 g/d
Gemfibrozil (Lopid)	Muscle pain, several GI side effects including nausea and abdominal discomfort, skin rash (rare)	600 mg bid
Lovastatin (Mevacor) Pravastatin	Sleep disturbances, muscle pain syndrome	Starting 20 mg/d; range 40–80 mg/d; 10–40 mg
Niacin	Skin flushing, itching, GI upset	Starting 100–250 mg/d or bid; range 2–6 g/d; usually 2.0–4.5 g/d
Probucol (Lorelco)	Diarrhea, nausea, flatulence	500 mg bid

Key: **HDL**, high-density lipoproteins; **HMG-CoA**, 3-hydroxy-3-methylglutaryl-coenzyme A; **LDL**, low-density lipoproteins; **VLDL**, very-low-density lipoproteins.

NOTE: Reprinted by permission from *Patient Care*, February 15, 1989, p. 48.

NOTE: Gemfibrozil information adapated with permission from information appearing in *NEJM*, from Helsinki Heart Study. Primary-prevention trial with gemfibrozil in middle-aged men with dyslipidemia. *N. Engl. J. Med*. 1987, 317: 1237–1245. The remainder of the table from Gotto, A.M., Jr., "Cholesterol: New Approaches to Screening Management," *Diagnosis* 1988, 10(1):52.

the body. They also stimulate the liver's production of receptors, which "catch" free LDL cholesterol in the blood and remove it from the body. Remember: Many people who have problems with elevated LDL cholesterol lack sufficient receptors to take cholesterol out of the bloodstream.

Drugs in this category include cholestyramine (Questran) and colestipol (Colestid). Side effects may involve constipation, bloating, and problems with hemorrhoids.

Fibrates. These drugs focus on getting rid of excess triglycerides (a neutral fat) in the blood. At the same time, they often reduce total and LDL cholesterol levels and raise the level of "good" HDL cholesterol.

Gemfibrozil (lopid) is one of the most commonly used fibrates to lower LDL cholesterol. Possible side effects include gastrointestinal symptoms, such as nausea and development of gallstones.

The new stimulators of LDL receptors. This new class of drugs directly stimulates the work of the LDL receptors, which pull or catch the "bad" cholesterol out of the bloodstream. One of the most popular of these drugs is lovastatin (Mevacor). Possible side effects include liver problems and muscle soreness. These side effects are unusual. Another of these drugs is pravastatin (Pravachol), which has been recently approved and made available. Simvastatin (Zocor) is also available.

In administering these or other cholesterol-influencing drugs, physicians are likely to use a kind of step-care therapy, of the type we discussed in the preceding high blood pressure chapter. In other words, they may try one drug, and if that doesn't work properly, they may substitute or add another. For example, common combinations of medications include niacin plus Questran, and gemfibrozil plus niacin. Many physicians feel that lovastatin (Mevacor) and pravastatin (Pravachol) are first choices in lowering total cholesterol and LDL cholesterol.

The considerations in trying different drugs are the same mentioned throughout this discussion of atherosclerosis. In particular, your doctor will try to find a drug or combination of drugs that (1) lowers the "bad" LDL cholesterol; (2) maintains or raises levels of "good" HDL cholesterol; and (3) has minimal side effects. He or she will, of course, appreciate your continued efforts to reduce the fats and cholesterol in your diet. There is no substitute for diet.

Special Groups Need ____ Special Attention____

In discussing the problems and solutions surrounding the cholesterol challenge, two important groups often are left out—the elderly and women. Yet by neglecting those groups as we try to communicate the facts about cholesterol, we may be helping to increase the eventual risk of these people for stroke.

The elderly. Physicians and lay people alike once assumed that when a person passed age fifty, there was little that could be done about vascular problems such as hardening of the arteries (atherosclerosis) or high blood pressure. Now, though, we know that a great deal *can* be done to lower the risks of vascular problems, including stroke, at almost *any* age.

Studies by Dr. David H. Blankenhorn and his colleagues of the University of Southern California School of Medicine showed that significant reductions in total cholesterol and LDL cholesterol could actually *reverse* and unclog the arteries. This result was achieved in participants aged forty to fifty-nine by lowering blood fats through a combination of colestipol and niacin. Later studies by Dr. Dean Ornish have demonstrated that going on a diet low in saturated fat may accomplish a similar regression of hardening of the arteries for many people.

Other recent investigations have found that men older than sixty-five with total cholesterol of 250 or higher are twice as likely to develop heart disease. While the effects of blood pressure reduction and the cessation of smoking yield almost immediate results in people whose life expectancy is about fifteen years, the impact of cholesterol lowering will typically show benefits only after several years of therapy. In any case, medication is indicated if the LDL level does not decrease after three to six months of a low-fat, low-cholesterol diet.

There is no evidence that lowering LDL is of value after age seventy-five, *nor* is there evidence that it will not do you any good. An overall assessment of the person's health status can help determine whether lowering LDL should be attempted.

Women. Although younger women are generally at low risk for vessel-blocking stroke, their risk rises when they use oral contraceptives or pass through menopause.

● ***Bonnie L., the thirty-year-old.*** Bonnie had her cholesterol checked at a health fair. She had been taking oral contraceptives for several years and had a total cholesterol level of 222.

In later consultation with her physician, Bonnie learned about the importance of the "good" HDL component. After another blood test, she was reassured to learn that her HDL cholesterol was quite high, at 73 mg/dl. This meant that her total cholesterol to HDL ratio was a very healthy 3.04. Also, the blood tests showed that her "bad" LDL cholesterol was only 128—which was in the range of 130 mg/dl or below, which placed her in a low-risk category for clogging of the arteries.

As a consequence of this consultation, Bonnie felt considerably better about her blood fat profile. Since she didn't smoke, she could continue to take her birth control medication.

● *Harriet, the sixty-two-year-old.* When Harriet went through menopause in her early fifties, she began to experience hot flashes and other uncomfortable symptoms. Perhaps more important, the declining ability of her body to produce estrogen naturally caused her blood cholesterol level to increase and her HDL cholesterol to decrease.

Specifically, her total cholesterol rose from about 198 before menopause to an average of 245 afterward. Just as significant, her "good" HDL cholesterol declined from 63 before menopause to 41 after menopause. To put this another way, her ratio of total cholesterol to HDL cholesterol rose from a healthy 3.14 to a risky 5.98 after menopause. (Remember: The upper end of the acceptable ratio for women is 4.50.)

To counter the "change of life" symptoms and also to put her blood fat profile into better balance, Harriet's physician placed her on estrogen replacement therapy. This means that her physician prescribed an estrogen-containing medication that provided her body with a significant part of the estrogen she had lost by going through menopause. Also, her physician prescribed progestin, a drug that is usually given with estrogen because estrogen alone may increase the risk of endometrial (womb) cancer.

As a result of this estrogen replacement therapy, Harriet M. experienced a resurgence of her HDL cholesterol and a lowering of her total cholesterol, owing primarily to a decrease in her "bad" LDL levels. During the year after she started this treatment, her total cholesterol declined from 245 mg/dl to 220—a figure that was higher than her premenopause measurement, but still acceptable in light of the increase in her HDL cholesterol. The HDLs rose from 41 to 62 as a result of the estrogen medication. The end result of her treatment was that her total cholesterol to HDL cholesterol ratio declined from 5.98 to 3.55. Harriet has managed to maintain this ratio up to her present age of sixty-two. As a consequence of these changes in her blood fats, her risk for stroke and heart attack has been reduced considerably. And most important, she feels better, too!

It should be evident from this discussion of the principles of lowering and adjusting blood cholesterol—and the various illustrations recounted—that it is usually possible for people to conquer the cholesterol challenge. Life-style changes, including alterations in diet and exercise habits, are often enough to do the trick. If necessary, a multitude of effective medications are also available.

I will even go so far as to say that *most* people now at risk for cardiovascular disease by clogged arteries should be able to reduce greatly or even eliminate that risk with the nutritional, fitness, and medical tools available. So don't wait a second longer: Meet the cholesterol and atherosclerosis and blood pressure challenge head-on!

Chapter Seven

The Stroke Victim's Survival Plan

When stroke actually strikes, the speed of response by the patient, the patient's family or friends, and the physician can be crucial to survival and recovery. Time is of the essence. This chapter will present a step-by-step "survival plan" to help stroke victims and their relatives and friends understand how response time needs to be speeded up to maximize the chance for recovery.

Unfortunately, medical practice hasn't demanded as quick a response for the stroke victim as for the heart attack victim. Within minutes of chest pain, an electrocardiogram can be conducted and treatment started to counter a heart attack. A current goal is to start definitive treatment for a heart attack within an hour. But with a stroke, it may take hours or even days for a patient to undergo a brain scan (such as a "computed tomography," or CT, scan). Yet effective treatment demands that such a scan be completed as quickly as possible.

If we don't seem to be moving quickly enough, it is because more red tape needs to be cut. Public attitudes need to be changed to encourage the public to demand more speed in the treatment of stroke victims. The public *must* be educated and respond if we hope to minimize brain damage owing to stroke.

A National Heart Attack Alert Program has been organized. A similar program for stroke is urgently needed.

When a stroke hits, the patient or family sometimes *waits* to call a physician; then *waits* for transport to the hospital; then *waits* to be admitted; then *waits* for an examination; then *waits* for a brain scan; then *waits* for treatment. The curse of waiting can seal the fate of a stroke victim.

As you read the following overview of the experience of the typical stroke victim, ask yourself, "How can I assist the medical staff to do its work better? Also, how can I ask the questions that may help preserve the health—and perhaps even save the life—of my loved one?"

_____Phase 1: The Diagnosis_____

Strokes strike quickly and usually inflict their greatest damage within minutes to a few hours of the onset of the attack. If the person experiencing the stroke returns to normal within less than twenty-four hours, the event is termed a "transient ischemic attack," or TIA, as described in Chapter Four. On the other hand, if the symptoms or signs last more than twenty-four hours, the incident is regarded as a completed stroke.

The physician will try to obtain a history of the events that preceded the stroke in order to discern clues as to the cause of the stroke. He or she will be particularly interested in whether the patient ever had a previous TIA. The physician will also, of course, be concerned about a history of hypertension, headaches, mental clarity, loss of consciousness, and weakness of the extremities. Finally, he will conduct the examination as expeditiously as possible.

Ultimately, the physician will want to use one of the brain scanning methods to confirm his initial diagnosis. For example, he may use computed tomography (CT scans) or nuclear magnetic resonance imaging (MRI or NMR). These approaches allow him actually to view a picture of the brain to assess the cause and extent of any damage.

However, immediate access to scanning machines may be limited, even in well-equipped urban areas. So the initial diagnosis during the first few minutes or hours following a stroke is likely to focus on history of events and outward signs.

Outward signs and symptoms of stroke due to vessel blockage. There are a number of specific types of stroke that result from a blockage of vessels leading to the brain, and each has its own peculiar characteristics. Here are a few that occur with many *blockage strokes:*

* Weakness or paralysis of the muscles of one or more extremities and change in sensation of the face, arms, or legs

* Weakness or paralysis in the upper and lower extremities of the same side

* Inability to speak properly

* Inability to understand speech

* Visual problems

* Rotation of the eyes or head toward the side of the brain affected

* Urinary incontinence

* Inability to maintain balance

* Mental confusion

Bleeding within the brain (an intracerebral hemorrhage) may have somewhat different symptoms:

* Headaches, which may be accompanied by nausea and vomiting

* Loss of consciousness or mental clarity

* Loss of muscle abilities and/or sensation in the right or left limbs

A *subarachnoid hemorrhage,* which may result from the bursting of a balloonlike nodule (aneurysm) in a vessel of the brain, will have features that are similar to the more common bleeding stroke. But there are a few variations. These symptoms usually occur as a "package" and are interrelated to one another:

* Headache, sometimes on one side or at the back of the head

* A stiff neck

* Nausea and vomiting

* Occasional visual problems

* Coma (in severe cases)

The physician will evaluate these signs and symptoms and will also consider the patient's past medical history. Among other things, he will focus on any previous heart disease or stroke in the patient or his close relatives, hypertension, diabetes, smoking habits, and other risk factors.

During the exam, he will order a variety of laboratory and scanning tests. When the results of these become available, he'll be able to confirm a diagnosis. In more detail, the testing possibilities include:

* Doppler sonography, or the use of sound waves to identify obstructions in the arteries in the neck going to the brain or arteries in the brain itself.

* A lumbar puncture of the spine. If the fluid is bloody, the likelihood is that the stroke has resulted from a hemorrhage. The procedure is being performed with much less frequency these days since the advent of brain scanning.

* A CT (computed tomography) scan. This technique involves placing the patient in a tubelike device so that the brain can be scanned with radiation. It produces slicelike pictures of the brain. If this procedure is conducted immediately after a stroke, bleeding in the brain will be evident in the CT picture. If the stroke has resulted from a clot that is blocking a vessel, it will typically take one to two

days for the problem to appear on the CT screen. So it is possible to confirm or eliminate a diagnosis of a brain hemorrhage immediately with a CT scan. But it takes longer to identify a blocked artery.

* Nuclear magnetic resonance imaging (MRI or NMR). With this method, the patient is placed in a scanner and exposed to a magnetic blast thirty thousand times stronger than the earth's magnetic field. Blockages of vessels leading to the brain can be picked up faster this way than through the CT scan. Hemorrhage is also evident on MRI scanning.

  Neither of these types of scanning is "invasive." This means that injections, dyes, or tubes inserted into the body are usually not necessary. The NMR requires that the patient enter headfirst into a circular, tubelike device. During the procedure, the device produces jackhammer sounds, which result from the magnetism needed to conduct the test. Explanations of what to expect and reassurance to the patient can avert a sense of claustrophobia that may occur. This procedure takes more time and needs more patient cooperation than a CT scan.

* Positron emission tomography (PET). This state-of-the-art technique involves surrounding the patient with a large ring that can detect energy from particles (positrons) emitted from the brain. A computer then processes this information and creates an image of blood flow in the brain. Unfortunately, PET machines aren't widely available; they are extremely expensive; and the precise value of this method in stroke patients is still academic presently.

After the physician has identified the type of stroke involved, he will focus on medical responses that are appropriate to the specific cause of the problem. Treatment is ongoing at this stage because certain measures must be taken immediately, and then more complex diagnostic tests have to be conducted.

Phase 2: The First Wave of Medical Responses
_____for _All_ Strokes_____

Just getting a patient to a hospital quickly presents practical problems. Distance from the hospital, availability of transportation, and traffic conditions are among the obstacles that need to be overcome. Rural, suburban, and urban sites each present special problems.

Once the patient has arrived at a hospital, it may take an hour or more to complete the admission procedure, much less get an examination and a brain scan. Although hospitals are trying to cut this time to a bare minimum, it has been estimated that it may take almost two hours from the onset of stroke symptoms at home to arrive at the hospital. Time is precious at this stage because brain cells are in peril.

Regardless of whether the cause of the stroke is vessel blockage or bleeding in the brain, the medical and nursing staffs will begin taking important steps on their first contact with the patient. The benefits of the science and art of nursing are very apparent in the management of the stroke victim. All efforts are focused on helping to maintain the vitality of brain tissue surrounding the injured tissue.

Among other things, the medical staff's responses will include the following:

* They will keep airways to the lungs open. Maintaining this airway is primary in the unconscious patient. Family and friends need to recognize the lifesaving value of "intubation." This procedure, which is sometimes necessary, involves the insertion of a breathing tube into the trachea, or windpipe, via the mouth. The device ensures that air and its vital oxygen content are being delivered to the patient.

* They will monitor the blood pressure. Fluctuations and variations in the blood pressure are related to the vital blood flow to the brain. Coping with the blood pressure

changes and maintaining the circulation are among the most important objectives of the staff.

∗ Any seizures must be stopped. Seizures, though uncommon with stroke, encourage additional damage to the brain tissue. Medications are often effective to head off seizures.

∗ Infections must be avoided to prevent pneumonia or urinary tract problems. Preventive measures will be taken.

∗ A precipitous drop in blood sugar is a danger in the initial stage of a stroke and may trigger mental confusion or a coma. Intravenous glucose may be required.

∗ Dehydration is a threat. In some cases, water and electrolytes will have to be administered to the patient, often through intravenous means. Nutritional requirements may be met orally or by tube (intravenous feedings).

The oxygen issue. The use of oxygen in the stroke victim may make the patient's family feel better but is unlikely to benefit the patient. Under most circumstances, oxygen administration does not affect the outcome because the oxygen-carrying power of the blood is already at its maximum.

On another front, attempts may be made to introduce more oxygen to the brain through the reduction of brain swelling after the stroke. Brain swelling (brain edema) is a feared complication of stroke because the swelling occurs in a rigid structure—the bony skull. Attempts to reduce brain swelling temporarily are performed by use of medications that act by extracting fluids. Examples of such medications are Mannitol and Glycerol. Other medications are being evaluated for this purpose.

When the nerve cell loses its supply of oxygen, chemical transmitters inside the cell leak out. These chemicals make matters worse. If it were possible to block the chemicals, the damage to the cell caused by a lack of oxygen could be limited. One of the many toxic chemicals liberated is called glutamate, and as a result, many glutamate blockers are being explored.

In the treatment of a heart attack or stroke, there is what

is called a "window of opportunity." That is the time in which it is thought that medication would be most effective. During that time, imaging with the CAT scanner or MRI will distinguish the presence of hemorrhage in the brain or the fact that the stroke is likely due to a blocked artery.

Currently we are targeting the first four hours as the window of opportunity with the realization that treatment within much less time approaches the ideal. If the window of opportunity were reduced to ninety minutes or less, the probability of greater improvement with treatment would be higher.

Phase 3: Special Treatment of Stroke Patients with Blockage of _____Arteries to the Brain_____

Most of the points mentioned in Phases 1 and 2 apply to the patient who has suffered a stroke as a result of the blockage of an artery to the brain. But there are some additional issues of special interest that relate to the treatment of this kind of stroke victim.

The use of TPA to restore blood flow to the brain.
TPA is the acronym for tissue plasminogen activator. It is a naturally occurring substance that has been genetically engineered and manufactured. TPA dissolves blood clots and has been approved and used successfully for the treatment of heart attacks.

Although TPA is still experimental in the treatment of stroke, the experience thus far indicates that blockage of blood to the brain can be dissolved and blood supply restored. An actual reversal of symptoms of stroke in some has been observed. The downside of the use of TPA is the increased risk of brain hemorrhage.

The thinking thus far is that if the patient can be treated with TPA within ninety minutes of a blockage-type stroke, the chances for recovery are good. With a longer interval between stroke onset and use of TPA, however, improvement is less likely to occur. Also, the risk of complications becomes greater.

More concerted efforts on the part of the public, paramedics, physicians, and hospital administrators is necessary to bring response time for stroke down to the heart attack response time. Actually, the response time for stroke should be even *faster* than that for a heart attack because the brain is even more sensitive to the lack of blood supply and does not have the circulatory reserves of the heart.

To sum up, then, an increasing number of studies are showing that TPA can be quite useful, and even lifesaving, when a first-line diagnosis makes it fairly certain that the stroke is the result of a blood clot. At the present time, the use of the drug with stroke victims is considered experimental and carries risks. For it to be used, patients or their next of kin must sign an approval and release form. A practical drawback is that it is being used only at medical centers widely dispersed across the country.

Most medical personnel you encounter will take these points into consideration as they begin to treat a stroke patient. They will be appreciative of your efforts to help reduce the response time at home and in the hospital. Recognition by all that speed is of the essence reflects the common goal—namely, the reduction of brain damage.

As more medications such as TPA become available (e.g., streptokinase), and as we learn how and when to use them, the focus will shift more and more toward emergency responses to stroke.

A cautionary word on surgery. There is no surgery that will *reverse* a stroke that has already occurred. When a stroke occurs from a blockage in one of the neck (carotid) arteries leading to the brain, a form of surgery known as "emergency carotid endarterectomy" has sometimes been performed in the past. This procedure involves scraping out the passageway and inner lining of the neck artery and removing any clot that may be present. But once the damage has been done, it cannot be reversed.

This type of surgery, as we have seen, can be of value in stroke prevention.

Special Treatment of a Stroke Patient with a Blocked Artery Resulting from a Traveling Clot (Embolism)

The backbone of treatment designed to prevent traveling clots, or "emboli," is the use of so-called blood thinners. Also known as anticoagulants, these medications may prevent a traveling clot.

If a stroke resulting from a traveling clot (embolism) is currently under way, physicians use medications to prevent other clots that may be heading toward the brain.

Carl T., for example, suffered a stroke from a traveling clot to the brain. Because he also suffered from an irregular heartbeat (auricular fibrillation) his physician feared that he might be one of the many people who were in danger of a second stroke. The reason: A heart problem such as his is known to be a source of traveling clots (emboli).

Before giving him the anticoagulant medication, Carl's physician determined from brain scans that there was no bleeding in his brain. The physician then gave him the drug called heparin initially. It was followed by another clot-preventing drug, warfarin (Coumadin). He has had no other stroke occurrences.

There are about one million people with auricular fibrillation who can be considered candidates for anticoagulant therapy. It is estimated that 100–150 strokes per day could be prevented by such therapy!

The two medications that are in current use to delay clotting are (1) the old familiar effective standby, aspirin; and (2) warfarin (Coumadin). Heparin is reserved for in-hospital use because it is not effective when administered orally.

Special Treatment of a Stroke Patient with Bleeding in the Brain

With a patient who has suffered a stroke from bleeding in the brain, the major objectives are to control and stop the hemorrhaging, and to prevent rebleeding. Toward this end, several responses may be appropriate. The first category involves nonsurgical, medical treatments; the second, surgery.

The nonsurgical response. Lydia S., a seventy-two-year-old retiree, suffered a stroke as a result of a ruptured vessel in her brain resulting from high blood pressure. The blood spread over part of her brain tissue causing the formation of a clot known as a hematoma. (Just a thimbleful of blood can cause a hematoma.)

She was treated as described in Phases 1 and 2 in this chapter. At this early stage, her physician ascertained that she was not taking any anticoagulants before the stroke occurred.

Among the problems the physician faced was the unanswered question of when and how much to lower Lydia's blood pressure. Lowering the blood pressure the right amount can help prevent further hemorrhaging and hasten recovery. But lowering it too much can have serious adverse effects, such as hypotension (blood pressure that is too low to sustain good flow of blood to the brain).

Using antihypertensive medications, which are commonly employed for many stroke patients with a brain hemorrhage, the physician succeeded in lowering the pressure just the right amount. Consequently, Lydia's condition stabilized, and she began to recover.

When is surgery appropriate for strokes by hemorrhage? When it has been determined that stroke is due to hemorrhage in the brain, surgery is rarely indicated. Some patients make remarkable recoveries from such strokes without surgery, and surgery may entail dangers and difficulties for many bleeding stroke victims. But if the physicians determine that hemorrhage has occurred in the part of the brain that controls coordination (the cerebellum), successful surgery is a possibility.

Bleeding in the space between the brain and the membrane that covers the brain (the subarachnoid space) often occurs because of a burst aneurysm. An aneurysm is a weakness in the walls of the artery that gradually balloons and may eventually burst. Surgery is necessary to "clip off" the aneurysm or repair the burst vessel and prevent further bleeding. These "subarachnoid hemorrhages" cause about 5–10 percent of all stroke.

With the advent of microsurgical techniques, which can be used to stabilize and treat complications of subarachnoid hemorrhage, the outlook for this problem has much improved. The recovery of these critically ill patients depends on the combined skills of the neurosurgeon and the critical care staff.

AVMs—arteriovenous malformations—are coiled masses of arteries and veins that are congenital in origin. They are situated on the surface of the brain and usually cause no problems unless they bleed. The most frequent age for this type of bleeding to occur is between fifteen and thirty years. There are several different methods of treatment that are usually quite effective. These treatments range from surgery to radiation therapy.

More on the _____Surgery Solution_____

What does surgery have to offer to *prevent* a future stroke? As with many other aspects of treating a stroke patient, there is a difference of medical opinion. But here are some general rules of thumb that are accepted by many physicians and researchers.

Opening up and cleaning out the neck arteries (a procedure known as a carotid endarterectomy) is often used when X rays of the blood vessels (angiogram) have shown that a carotid artery is significantly clogged. Recent guidelines indicate that surgery is appropriate to scrape out a blocked artery when the vessel is more than 70 percent shut off by plaque. On the other hand, if the blockage (occlusion) is *less* than 70 percent, medical treatment, such as aspirin or other clot preventers, is an alternative.

Many times, physicians also will limit surgical operations to patients who have some symptoms, such as a transient ischemic attack (TIA) or a mild stroke that permits full recovery. Doctors often will *not* operate if the patient has other serious health problems, such as kidney, heart, or lung failure;

unstable diabetes mellitus; unregulated high blood pressure; or cancer that carries a poor prognosis.

"Star Wars" surgery. Some new developments on the surgery horizon hold great promise for the future—though currently they carry risks. One of these is the use of a cyclotron to shoot helium ions at high speeds into the brain to destroy malformed vessels—the arteriovenous malformations (AVMs) that are in danger of bursting.

These abnormal arteries and veins have been referred to as "time bombs" in the brain. They can rupture or leak, causing a serious stroke. Because the risk of *not* operating seems more significant than the risk of using the new technology, this procedure may be recommended for some patients.

In a Stanford University Medical Center study, 80 percent of more than forty patients experienced "excellent or good results" with the technology—and the threat of stroke was greatly reduced.

In the Days, Weeks, and Months _____Following a Stroke_____

It is a mistake to view a stroke as a one-time event. In fact, a stroke is a health threat that should be placed on a continuum of danger and concern.

First of all, there's a high risk that one stroke will be followed by a second, especially if the cause of the first was a traveling blood clot, or embolism. The existence of one stroke is a warning that conditions exist that predispose the patient to another stroke. Anticlot medications may be administered to help prevent a recurrence.

The Depression Problem

After the patient passes through the first week or two of recovery, there is a great likelihood that depression will set in. In fact, nearly 50 percent of all stroke survivors suffer from some degree of depression within a few months of their stroke.

That response is quite understandable. A relatively healthy person before the stroke, the victim becomes aware of a number of physical limitations. He has become dependent against his will, or cannot do what he did before. So a reactive depression is understandable.

One problem with depression is that the "low" attitude of the patient may inhibit the motivation and will necessary for a fast recovery and rehabilitation. So physicians, friends, and family of a stroke victim should be alert to the onset of any depression and make every effort to counter it.

What are the signs that depression may be present? Typically, the patient will display sadness, irritability, a sense of inadequacy, and pessimism about the future. Also, there may be a loss of appetite, an inability to sleep, and a marked decrease in energy.

One cause of the depression is often an emotional response to the loss of mobility or health. To help the patient, friends and family members can encourage discussion of these losses and provide a support network. They should also urge the patient to begin a "comeback" by recapturing some of his old muscular and mental abilities.

There may also be biological causes of the depression that result from the damage to the brain inflicted by the stroke. Memory, emotions, and other mental functions can be directly affected by the stroke. Many times, a very severe depression will lift as the brain centers triggering the depression heal. In a number of cases, however, antidepressant medications will have to be employed to relieve the symptoms of depression.

These poststroke considerations, including the pervasive depression that hits many patients, are extremely important to keep in mind as we move to our next topic—the rehabilitation of the stroke victim.

Chapter Eight

You Can Come Back!

The results of a stroke can be devastating; damage to the brain may cause a loss of:

* muscle power and control

* speech

* vision

* thinking ability

* a variety of other human functions

Yet the effects of the injury can often be minimized and recovery of many or even most of the lost abilities may become possible—*if* the stroke victim and his family and friends respond appropriately to the crisis. In short, if you have a stroke, in many cases *you can come back*, provided you devise and follow a wise action plan for recovery.

Worst-Case and
_____Best-Case Scenarios_____

To understand the possibilities, as well as the pitfalls, of the aftermath of a stroke, consider these two scenarios, which are based on the experiences of actual patients. The first person, the "worst case," could have had a relatively happy and productive life, but he and his loved ones fell into several common traps. The second person came closer to realizing his full potential to bounce back.

The worst case. Norman A., a fifty-eight-year-old divorced man, had always been a difficult person. He was the father of three adult, highly intellectual children, but he couldn't get along with them. He always had to have his own way, and as a result, he lived alone in a studio apartment and rarely saw his two sons and daughter.

Then, he suffered a stroke, which crippled his right side and resulted in great speech problems. Still, both his physicians and family thought he might be able to improve with the proper motivation and opportunities for rehabilitation. But after eight weeks of attempts by both family members and doctors to get him on the road to improvement, he was still lying in bed without the ability to speak clearly, feed himself, or move about.

The medical staff agreed that his "brain is all right." Furthermore, by every indication he had the capacity to improve. But he didn't.

What went wrong?

As the family and physicians began to piece the picture together, they concluded that Norman had become completely bitter about the experience and, in effect, had given up on life. He didn't like his children or other relatives; he had no close friends; and from all appearances, he didn't like the medical staff either. On occasion, he would push or even bat nurses and physicians away with his good hand when they got near him.

Finally, Norman developed pneumonia several times, and even his unaffected left side grew weaker. His family now realizes that there is little hope that he will improve, and they are looking for a nursing facility for him. Norman will undoubtedly let his displeasure be known and blame his children, and a legacy of guilt will descend on their shoulders.

In short, Norman's weaknesses and unlovable qualities during his healthy days were magnified by his stroke. As a result, he failed to take advantage of any opportunities for improvement.

The best case. Arnold M., a thirty-eight-year-old salesman, suffered a stroke that impaired his ability to speak, walk, and use his right side. Specifically, he had some difficulties finding words during conversations; he couldn't write well with his right hand; and at first, he couldn't get around on his feet.

But Arnold was motivated to get better. He had been a top sales rep, and he wanted to retrieve some of those skills of persuasion that he had once enjoyed. After a few weeks of therapy, he was able to walk with a cane, and he started learning how to write with his left hand.

After the completion of his stay in the hospital and the rehabilitation center, he went home to live with his parents. There, he continued to improve. Now, he can walk without a cane, has an apartment of his own, and has resumed his relationships with girlfriends.

Arnold is still trying to find the right vocational fit, but this is an exciting time in his life. He has recovered most of his mental and physical capacities, and is now considering a new profession, perhaps one related to helping other stroke victims with their rehabilitation.

Clearly, Arnold has snapped back much more successfully from his stroke than Norman—and the reasons are fairly obvious. Arnold's younger age contributed to his flexibility and motivation. Arnold was more inclined to take advantage of the rehabilitative opportunities that were available. Additionally, he had good personal and family relationships, which provided him with essential support in those first days after the stroke and the hospital stay. In short, there is often a good chance for a stroke victim to come back, if only he or she can understand and take advantage of the possibilities.

The Basics
of Rehabilitation

Every stroke victim and the friends and family members of the victim must keep the major goals and principles of rehabilitation in mind. These are as follows:

1. The motor, speech, cognitive, and other impaired functions need to be improved. Whatever has been damaged should be targeted for repair!

2. Although they may not be able to be fully restored, the mental and social capacities of patients should be adapted to more limited functioning, so as to help the patient achieve the maximum independence and satisfying relationships.

3. Wherever possible, the patient should be returned to the activities of his or her normal daily life.

There is obviously a premium on starting rehabilitation and recovery quickly because the longer the patient waits, the more time begins to work against him. A number of experts have summed up this point and other basic principles of rehabilitation this way:

Begin early.

Be systematic.

Build up in stages.

Focus on rehabilitation treatments that are designed specifically to help improve the particular disability. In other words, keep your priorities clearly in mind, and don't be distracted by trying for some sort of "general" improvement.

To give you a fuller picture of how these basics of rehabilitation work in more detailed, practical situations, I want to invite you to participate with me in an extended "conversation" on rehabilitation.* Common questions of stroke victims and their families will be posed, and then, in the voice of a composite "rehabilitation expert," answers will be forthcoming. Further, specific details on rehabilitation techniques can be found in the Appendix.

A Conversation
_____on Rehabilitation_____

Q. What do you mean when you refer to the "recovery" of a stroke patient?

A. I'm not happy with the word "recovery," mainly because of the way it can be misunderstood by patients and family members. To me, a recovery is a return of function so that the patient can be reintegrated into an acceptable life-style. Very often, however, the patient or the family defines recovery as a return to the condition that the patient was in before the stroke occurred—even if a full return of functioning isn't possible.

So when I hear the term recovery, it somehow rings alarms of concern because I fear the family or the patient will not be realistic. It is therefore my job to teach the patient and also the family what is realistic in terms of their joint goals.

Q. At what stage of the stroke illness would you, as a rehabilitation expert, want to see the patient?

A. I like to see the patient as soon as possible, preferably within a week after the stroke. Then, I can recommend at the earliest stage how to follow through on the disability. The problems may vary from a speech difficulty to complete "dissection," or disability of an entire side of the body. One half of the person may be completely gone—and so it's necessary to begin to work on the impairment as quickly as possible.

*Much of this "conversation" has been taken from a conversation I had with Dr. Valery Lanyi of the renowned Rusk Institute.

Q. What is the role of the primary care physicians?

A. I rely on support from the primary care physician since many of the patients have associated illness such as high blood pressure, heart disease, or diabetes.

Also, in the rehabilitation unit, I direct the therapy with the knowledge that I have the backup of the primary care physician.

Q. What are the implications of neglecting the unaffected side of the body?

A. Every effort must be made to engage the unaffected side. Even when there is a return of some function on the impaired side, the stroke victim may not take full advantage of that recovery if his strong side isn't in good shape. The return of strength and sensation doesn't necessarily mean that the person can fully use the damaged part of his body. So the stronger side often plays a crucial role in supporting and improving the weaker side.

A form of denial may also occur where the patient assumes he is incapable of any improvement. Everyone—the physician, the family, and the patient—must work hard to fight that denial.

Q. Suppose you have a weak or flaccid left side. What do you do?

A. Move the limbs that aren't moving. Work on balance. Try to learn to sit and stand. It's remarkable how many patients can respond to efforts to stand up, even if they have undergone significant brain damage. But you must begin early, within a week or so after the stroke!

Preoccupation with the affected side by the patient and family can be counterproductive. Emphasis should be on the integration of the affected and unaffected sides.

Q. What are your main objectives in terms of teaching a patient how to do things again?

A. It's a matter of survival. The stroke patient should first learn to feed himself. Some patients lose their gag reflex, and they can't handle independent eating. But most are able to deal with this.

Then, the next most important thing is to be independent in bathroom activities. The objective is to maximize function.

Q. How important is it to learn how to walk again?

A. For most patients and families it's very important—but I'm not sure it should be. Sometimes, it's the hardest thing to explain to a high-powered intellectual that the energy he or she expends in walking would be better used in sitting in a mobile wheelchair and using the brain!

For example, one business executive suffered a left-sided stroke. He tried and tried to walk again, but all to no avail. Neither he nor his family was ever able to recognize that if he had been content just to sit in a wheelchair, he could have had a very satisfying life. He could have joined a study group; he could have begun writing by dictating into a tape recorder; he could have spent time reading; or he could have learned to enjoy music.

Instead, he became depressed because his disability, which included a severe lack of balance, prevented him from walking. This kind of situation is a tragedy because the patient and his family fail to recognize what a wonderful quality of life is possible if only the disabilities are approached realistically.

Q. Rehabilitation is often a slow, step-by-step process. Can you elaborate?

A. A physical therapist, occupational therapist, and others on the rehabilitation team will work gradually on the patient's range of motion of the affected limbs. That means that even if the person can't move an arm at first, it will be moved for him. Also, the *uninvolved* side of the body will be strengthened. That enhances overall support and functioning of the body.

If there is a swallowing problem, we'll lead the person step-by-step via repeated swallowing tests under X-ray control. In sequence, he'll learn to take in thin liquids, thick liquids, thin solids, and thick solids.

Another important part of the rehabilitation process is working on balance. We want our patients to be able to sit up and then to stand, if possible. If they are able to walk, great! But the process often occurs in several stages. First, they learn to stand by themselves. Then, they begin to move about, using an aid, such as a walker, a quad-cane, or a regular cane.

Reestablishing coordination and bilateral hand activities are among the chief objectives. Occupational therapists work in painstaking detail on eye-hand coordination, as well as on strengthening and retraining the muscles.

We'll also focus on improving facial muscles and speech therapy. The goal is to help the patient return to a normal daily life.

Q. What's the biggest problem you have with patients?

A. Probably the worst thing is that the stroke patient wants desperately to do some favorite activity but he can't. Frustration and depression will result if he can't get a grip on this drive or need.

Q. What kinds of problems do family members and friends face?

A. Too often, they want recovery to occur too rapidly. They think that if the patient just exercises enough, he'll get better. But they don't realize that some people will never recover certain functions. Also, they fail to understand how tired and exhausted a stroke can make a person.

Although we want to start rehabilitation as soon as possible, there is a danger in starting it too early, when the patient is still exhausted from the physical trauma. It's like being in a major auto accident. You have to rest awhile before you can really begin recovery.

Q. If you could give the families of stroke victims one piece of advice, what would it be?

A. Allow the patient to be independent. Find devices, such as button buttoners or bottle openers that allow him to do things for himself. Also, make time to let the patient finish a task. If you have to get to an appointment in ten minutes, then perhaps you'll have to dress him. Otherwise, take an extra half hour and let him dress himself.

Also, arrange for the patient to do as many chores around the house as possible. The more cooking, cleaning, and other tasks he can complete, the more confidence he'll gain and the more his mood will improve.

Q. *What can be done for a patient who doesn't have a family available to help?*

A. It's important for every person who is alone to get involved in some kind of support group. Unfortunately, if the disabilities or medical problems are relatively severe, the individual will probably have to go immediately into a nursing home, where rehabilitation efforts may be minimal. Whenever possible, the isolated patient should try to secure twenty-four-hour help by a person trained in rehabilitation exercises and techniques.

Q. *Describe how a rehabilitation team might work.*

A. The patient spends most of his time in the hospital with the nurses. They are the ones who care for the intimate aspects of daily life, the hygiene, the administering of medications, and the other necessities.

First, the nurses on the team might become involved in helping with bladder control and bowel training. In addition to standard nursing duties, they would also dress the patient, help him sit up, and assist him in eating.

Then, there is the physical therapist, who works on helping the person move his affected limbs and also helps him move about and walk. In addition, the physician may order orthostes [braces]. The therapist will work with the patient and teach him to walk with the brace. These orthostes are devices that work against gravity to help the person stand or sit without other assistance. It's a question of safety, as well as mobility. If an affected foot drops down at the wrong moment, the patient could trip over it and be severely hurt in a fall.

A speech therapist will be involved in hearing and speech evaluation. She will assist the patient in expressing himself and also assist the other staff members in communicating and working better with the victim. Emphasis is on short sentences and simple speech. A flexible program is vital. The result can be highly rewarding.

Q. *What about recreation?*

A. A recreational therapist is often another member of the team. On Friday nights and the weekends, life in a hospital or other medical facility can be depressing. So the person in charge of recreation will help the patient find a card game, go to a movie, do horticulture therapy, or just get outside in the fresh air. The art of recreation is fast becoming a science.

Q. *Is there any way to avoid depression after a stroke?*

A. The absence of depression after a stroke is pathology! It's unnatural! Nobody in this situation should sit around with a big smile on his face and say, "Hello, I just had a stroke, and I feel great!" That's abnormal. Reactive depression is normal, and most patients will pull out of it in a few weeks.

Q. *How do you motivate patients to want to improve?*

A. You first find out what is most important to them and then begin to deal with that. You try to find that spring or button that makes them want to deal with their problem.

But in communicating with stroke victims, you must not condescend to them. It's important to deal with them exactly as you would have before the accident. Still, there is an enormous amount of prejudice toward the disabled in terms of talking down to them.

Q. *Are the various assisting devices really helpful for stroke patients?*

A. Absolutely. They can make a person totally independent. With the right devices, he or she can get dressed, turn a page, peel a potato, get on and off the toilet, and in general lead a full life. There are stocking putter-oners, shoe-taker-offers, button-hookers, motorized tricycles called scooters, and motorized wheelchairs. Many stroke victims can function quite well in a fully electrically operated environment.

Q. *How long does it take to figure out how far a person can go with rehabilitation?*

A. You can tell in two to three months. If a person doesn't go anywhere in the first six weeks, that's a bad sign. Only surprises happen after that.

Q. *How do you integrate the family into the rehabilitation process?*

A. I try to level with the family at the beginning. I say, "We are not God, and so we can't promise a return to full health." But I also tell them we will do the best we can for the patient. And I encourage family members to get involved in family groups at the hospital.

Q. *How can you tell if a stroke patient is ready to drive a car?*

A. At many facilities, there is a person who does nothing but take people out to check on their ability behind the wheel, including their reaction times.

I had a terrible time with one lawyer who had suffered a minor stroke. He insisted on going out driving while I insisted on his being thoroughly tested—because I knew that on his first attempts to drive, he had made enormous mistakes. He had a minor visual field defect, but that could have caused a major accident out on the road. It was a real struggle, but I finally succeeded in talking him out of driving himself.

Q. *How do a patient and family go about selecting a rehabilitation center?*

A. If the patient is in a hospital, the social worker there should be able to assist. It's best to go to a place that is recommended to you by your physician. If possible, it should be geographically available to relatives and friends so that visiting doesn't entail traveling great distances.

Q. *What does rehabilitation cost?*

A. Costs vary, depending on the part of the country. But to give you an idea, in one major urban area, the average is about $24,000 for thirty days in a semiprivate room and $27,000 to $28,000 for a private room. Doctor's fees are extra. Health insurance plans are important. Unfortunately, they usually don't cover all costs, and they vary considerably in expense and coverage.

Q. *How about some final advice about rehabilitation for families of stroke victims?*

A. It's good for the family to schedule events during the patient's hospitalization that are not disability-oriented. Take the person out to a movie, lunch, or somewhere else. Get your loved one out into the outdoors if possible.

Also, don't assume that the costliest benefits are necessarily the best. For example, you can spend a fortune on a full-time rehabilitation expert. Or you can hire an untrained but concerned and warm companion and *train* him or her how to help with recovery.

In one situation, a lovely young woman without any specialized training was taught to walk with the patient, help her dress, and otherwise assist in daily activities. Whenever you see the two of them on the street, the young woman is always smiling and encouraging. Those are qualities that you can't get by acquiring a degree or certificate at a university.

Chapter Nine

Decade of the Brain

As you have read this book, one or more of these questions were probably on your mind:

* How can I help with rehabilitation for a family member who has had a stroke?

* How can I prepare to respond to a loved one who has already had one stroke—and is at high risk for another?

* How can I take steps to prevent a stroke, since we have a family history of this problem?

I hope that as you have explored these pages, the answers to these and other pressing concerns have emerged. Many of the topics we've dealt with have involved descriptions of complex biological processes, medical procedures, and drug prescriptions. Yet to grasp the full meaning of what happens during the various types of strokes—and to understand what to do before, during, and after the trauma—it is necessary to do some hard, in-depth thinking.

At this point, you have the latest information available on

what can be done about stroke, but I realize there are still many unanswered questions. For example:

* What is the future outlook for TPA, the drug that is now being used for heart patients but isn't generally employed with stroke victims? Will it become more prevalent for those who have suffered an artery-blocking stroke, or will another, newer medication come along to replace it? Will we learn when and how to use it?

* What preventive medications will appear in the next few years to lower the risk of those who are most likely to suffer a stroke?

* What new rehabilitation techniques or prosthetic devices will make the lives of stroke victims easier?

* Will space-age diagnostic tools greatly reduce the response time of physicians who have to treat a stroke?

* What public health steps will be taken to increase the speed of getting the stroke victim to the hospital and into the hands of those who can care for him and make rapid, accurate decisions regarding treatment?

To spur further research and to improve the response capacities of the medical establishment, the National Institute of Neurological and Communicative Disorders and Stroke (NINCDS) has designated the 1990s as the Decade of the Brain. The outlook is bright because so much progress has been made in just the last ten years. Here are some observations by those at the NINCDS:

* Ten years ago, we were aware of only a few neurotransmitters, those chemical message carriers in the brain. Now, we have identified more than forty.

* Ten years ago, we were just beginning to use sophisticated DNA technology to determine the genetic components of brain disease. Today, there are almost too many scientific findings for the average physician to keep up with!

* Ten years ago, we thought it was impossible to replace or repair neurons damaged by trauma or disease. Today, we know that damaged neurons can grow back and transmit impulses again.

So plenty of progress has been made, and the prospects are bright for the next ten years. The explosion of information and treatment possibilities for the stroke patient promises that this progress will continue—at an accelerated pace.

What can *you* do to make the best practical use of all this forward movement in preventing, diagnosing, treating, and rehabilitating the ravages of stroke?

First, I'd suggest you use this book as a starting point. The basics are here, but the promise of future developments should inspire you to go beyond these pages and keep abreast of the latest breakthroughs. Clip reports in your local newspaper or in national magazines. Send away for new publications put out by information centers. Do your own research during the forthcoming years, as new strategies and responses to stroke become available, and the Decade of the Brain will become a time that can make you and your loved ones safer and healthier.

The leadership of the National Institute of Neurological and Communicative Disorders and Stroke (NINCDS) has served the nation well in organizing and coordinating research and teaching about stroke and its prevention.

Appendix A

Recovering from a Stroke

The American Heart Association has excellent publications available on stroke. They may be obtained by requesting them from the American Heart Association National Center, 7320 Greenville Avenue, Dallas, Texas 75231. The following excerpts are from a booklet entitled *Recovering from a Stroke*.

Bathing

When you bathe, take soap, washcloths and towels to the tub or shower area. Set the temperature of the water so it's not too hot or cold. Before you get in, test the water's temperature on your wrist (use your good wrist if the other one lacks feeling), or ask someone to test it for you.

Getting in and out of a wet, slippery tub can be dangerous, so be careful. It's a good idea to place non-skid tape on the bottom of the tub or shower and to install grab bars to make movement easier. You can attach a hand-held shower head to the faucet to make bathing underarms and private areas easier. Other aids, such as long-handled brushes and mittens with straps, can also help you bathe yourself. A word of caution:

Don't leave wet washcloths, towels, soap or lotions on the edge of the tub or in the shower.

You shouldn't be left alone in the shower or bathtub until you're fully recovered. Even when you're able to bathe alone, someone should be nearby to help. Keep a bell handy or have another means of calling for help.

Showers are safer than tub baths, because the openings make it easier to move in a shower. If standing in a shower makes you tired, try sitting on a chair. If you decide to put a chair in the shower, put suction cups on the legs so they won't slip.

If you don't have a shower and must use a tub, be very careful. Stores selling medical equipment have special seats that can be put on the rim of the tub—consider buying one. Another option is to use two chairs, sawing part of the legs off so the chairs are even with the rim of the tub. The chairs should be side-by-side and should face in the same direction, with one chair in the tub and the other next to the tub. Put suction cups on the legs so they won't slip. If you don't have chairs to use around the bathtub, have a strong person help you get in and out of the tub, and be very careful.

When you're climbing into the tub, step in with your weaker side first. When you're getting out of the tub, step out with your stronger side first. Before you climb out of the tub, though, dry your stronger arm and the tub edge so you won't lose your grip. Leaving the water in the tub until after you've climbed out is also a good idea—the buoyancy will help you get out.

Once you're out of the tub or shower, dry yourself completely and gently rub on a lotion to prevent your skin from drying out.

Dressing

There are some things you can make or buy that will make dressing easier. A few such items are:

* rings or strings on zipper pulls
* Velcro closures
* elastic waistbands
* snaps and grippers
* elastic shoelaces or other simple shoe closures

* stocking/sock spreaders (these can be made from old X-ray film)

* button hooks

Other articles besides those mentioned can also make your life easier. Pre-tied ties and elastic, front-hook brassieres are just two examples. Several companies now manufacture clothes made especially to be easy to put on. Sears is one place to buy such clothing.

Buttoning buttons, snapping snaps or tying shoelaces can be difficult. You'll have to relearn how to do these things a step at a time. You might, for example, practice buttoning a piece of clothing while it's on your lap. After you've learned how to do that, buttoning clothing you're wearing will be easier. You may find it's easier to put on your socks or shoes or tie your shoelaces if you put your foot on a footstool or box first.

For additional suggestions, consult an occupational therapist.

Eating

Chewing and swallowing food may be a problem for some people after they've had a stroke. It isn't uncommon for one or both sides of a person's mouth to lack feeling. If swallowing is hard for you or you sometimes begin choking, mention this to your doctor or therapist.

If eating is a problem for you, here is some advice:

Put only a small amount of food in your mouth at a time, and put it on the stronger side of your mouth. This will make swallowing easier and help prevent choking. Another point: Clear your mouth and throat after each bite of food, because there will be a tendency for food to become lodged in the weaker side of your mouth. You can check for trapped food with a mirror and remove it with your tongue or fingers. Clearing your throat after each bite of food is another way to prevent choking.

Some foods are easier to eat than others. Soft foods such as applesauce, hot cereal and sherbet, for example, are easier to swallow than liquids.

Breaking down foods in a blender is another way to make them easier to swallow. A number of department stores and health food stores sell small, portable blenders that work very well. A staff dietitian at a local health department can give you added help in choosing healthful, easy-to-eat foods.

As you recover, you can gradually return to a regular diet low in animal fat and cholesterol. Some people may have to reduce their intake of calories, sodium or both.

Some people who've had a stroke may have problems reaching for and spilling food, cutting meat, buttering bread, or opening containers. If you have these problems, don't get discouraged. It takes time, patience and practice to master these activities. Special items like those pictured above may help. An occupational therapist may be able to suggest other useful items.

Seeing

Several visual problems commonly occur after a stroke, and any of them may make it hard for you to do your daily tasks. You may have to practice your tasks over and over before you can do them properly.

With a loss of visual field, when you're looking straight ahead you may be unable to see things on your affected side. And if you've lost feeling on that side too, you may lose your awareness of that (weaker) side of your body. As a result, you may ignore objects placed on that side, have trouble reading, or dress only one side of your body and think you're completely dressed. As you move around, you also may bump into furniture or door frames. So you won't neglect your weaker side, train yourself to turn your head and look toward this side. Your friends can also remind you to turn your head toward your affected side.

If your stroke has affected your vision, some objects may look closer or farther away than they really are. This problem will probably be most apparent when you're trying to eat or dress, because you may over- or under-reach for an object. It also may cause you to bump into objects while walking.

Here are some ways to learn to judge distance more accurately:

1. At meals, consciously think about which foods and objects are close, far away, or middle-distance; also, think about "what is next to what."

2. Fold small laundered items and put them in a pile on your affected side.

3. When going up and down stairs, feel the height of the step with your foot before you shift your weight. Have someone with you to support you on your weaker side.

If it's hard to find an object in a cluttered drawer, or to see a white button on a white shirt, do the following:

* Sort the laundry and stack things neatly in drawers.

* Find the sleeve and neck openings on your clothing.

* Play simple card games or do puzzles that will help you remember what you see.

* Have someone sew buttons on your clothing that contrast with the color of the fabric; also use contrasting dishes on the table, etc.

* Place items you use a lot where they're easy to reach; keep them in uncluttered storage areas.

Special Equipment

Braces, splints or special equipment may be prescribed for different reasons. A leg brace or arm sling may give support; a wrist splint may prevent deformity; a spoon with a special handle may replace lost ability. If such equipment is prescribed for you, ask when it should be used and for how long. Also ask how to use and care for it.

* Check your equipment regularly to make sure it works properly and meets your needs.

* Keep using braces or splints until your doctor or therapist tells you to stop.

* There are many different kinds of wheelchairs. Your doctor, physical therapist or nurse will tell you the best kind

of wheelchair for you based on your size, method of transfers, life-style and other factors.

★ Safety, durability, portability, ease of maintenance and attractiveness are important features to consider in selecting a wheelchair.

★ Don't assume you'll have to buy an expensive one-hand-drive wheelchair just because your stroke affected one of your sides. If you're reasonably strong and can use one arm and leg, you can learn to guide a wheelchair using one hand and foot together.

Sexuality

People who were sexually active before having a stroke usually continue to be interested in sex afterward. Sometimes, however, they neglect or avoid sexual expression. Tension, emotional conflict or other problems can result.

Resuming a sexual relationship after a stroke may require changes. Weakness or paralysis, changes in body awareness, loss of feeling and speech problems can all interfere with sex. Then too, the frustration and embarrassment that often follows a stroke can reduce your self-esteem and further affect your sexual life. Finally, the stress of relearning how to perform daily tasks may cause you to be too tired for sex.

Depending on the area of the brain affected, a stroke can cause physical and emotional changes that affect a person's sex life. Men, for example, may have difficulty getting an erection or ejaculating. Similarly, a woman's vagina may have less feeling or less lubrication. Medication can also cause changes that make having sex more difficult.

Of course, while all these problems are possible, don't necessarily assume you'll have them. Everyone is different. If your sexual relationship with your partner has been affected, or you have questions about sexual activity, have a frank talk with your doctor or a qualified counselor or sex therapist.

Here are some other suggestions:

1. To maintain sexual interest, stay as attractive as you can through grooming and personal hygiene.

2. Share your feelings honestly and openly with your partner. Discuss your sexual interest and changes you need to make because of the limitations imposed by your stroke.

3. Ideally, plan for sexual activity in advance, just as you'd plan any other activity you wanted to enjoy to the fullest. The hours when you and your partner are most rested are the best: avoid times when you or your partner are exhausted from a heavy slate of activities. If possible, rest before having sex, allow plenty of time for lovemaking, and minimize distractions and interruptions.

4. A warm bath, pleasant music or a massage before lovemaking may help you relax and enjoy yourself more.

5. Be realistic about your physical abilities and disabilities. You and your partner may have to change your usual position in sex. Find a comfortable position that supports your weaker side and conserves your energy.

6. Using a water soluble, sterile lubricant may make penetration easier. Don't use petroleum jelly: It doesn't dissolve in water and can cause vaginal infection.

7. You and your partner may want to concentrate on alternatives to sexual intercourse such as hugging, kissing, caressing, touching or massaging. Touching can become a very important way for you and your partner to express your love for one another.

Driving

Before you try to drive, get clearance from your doctor. If your doctor says it's okay for you to drive, contact your State Department of Motor Vehicles and ask which requirements apply to you. It's possible you'll have to take a new road test, pass a driver's education course and install special equipment in your car. Do not, repeat, *do not* jeopardize your life and the lives of others by trying to drive before your doctor has given you permission.

If you need retraining, be sure you have a qualified instructor. To learn more about the various programs offered in your community, contact a rehabilitation center or an office of vocational rehabilitation in your area. Driver education programs are available in some communities.

_____Financial Support_____

If you need financial aid, food stamps or medical insurance, apply at your local Department of Social Services. You may also need equipment, nursing, a home health aide, rehabilitation therapy, a day care center, transportation, etc.

Medicaid is a form of medical insurance that can help you with these needs if you're eligible. Your eligibility is determined by guidelines based on your income and savings. If you want to apply for Medicaid, contact the Medicaid office in your local Department of Social Services.

Medicaid benefits vary widely from state to state. Your local Medicaid office can tell you about the benefits available in your state. You'll have to get a physician's written order to get the services you need.

Medicaid payments always go directly to the doctor or the person providing the service, so never pay for services yourself with the expectation of being reimbursed by Medicaid.

Medicare is another form of medical coverage that might help you. Under Medicare, unlike Medicaid, no financial guidelines have to be met. Eligibility is based on age (with the minimum age being 65) and the length of time a person has been disabled (with the minimum being two years).

In general, the home health services covered by Medicare are short-term, skilled services. These can be: occasional, part time, skilled nursing; physical therapy; speech therapy; and some occupational therapy and social work. Doctor's services and some equipment also are covered. Long-term maintenance isn't covered, except in certain states.

After you pay a $100 deductible per calendar year, Medicare will pay 80% of "reasonable charges" of covered services. You must pay the remaining 20% of "reasonable charges" and 100% of all charges in excess of what is defined as "reasonable." Benefits can be paid to your doctor or supplier, or they can be paid directly to you. To request benefits, submit a copy of the bill and a physician's prescription for the service to the Medicare office serving your area.

For more details about Medicare benefits, contact your local Social Security office or write to the Office of Health, Education and Welfare in Washington, D.C.

If you have private insurance, read your policy carefully or contact your insurance company to find out what services your policy covers.

Appendix B

Caring for a Person with Aphasia

The following excerpts are reprinted with the permission of the American Heart Association from the booklet *Caring for a Person with Aphasia.*

Introduction

At one time or another, we've all had trouble thinking of a word we wanted to say. Often it's someone's name, even a name we know well. Sometimes, especially when we most want to, we can't remember the name of a common object or concept. When these lapses occur occasionally, they're annoying. But for people with aphasia, they're frustrating facts of life.

Aphasia (a-FAY-zhia) is the name given to language problems caused by damage to the brain. Aphasia is a total or partial loss of the ability to use words. The most common cause of aphasia is stroke. Any disease or injury that damages brain tissue can cause aphasia, however. Not all strokes cause aphasia, but about 20 percent of people who have strokes suffer a serious loss of speech and language. The National Institutes of Health estimates that 85,000 new cases of aphasia occur every year, and that more than one million Americans have some form of aphasia.

_____What Is Aphasia?_____

To understand how a stroke can cause speech and language problems, and why so many different kinds of problems can occur, consider how speech and language are normally accomplished. Communication by speech isn't one event. It's made up of many different events that occur together or in stages.

Conveying a message requires you to think about what you want to say; to put your thought into the right words; then to say the words aloud. A similar series of events is necessary to understand what someone else says. First, you recognize that someone wants to tell you something. Once the person begins to talk, you must keep the words in mind. Then, even before the speaker stops, you must put together everything that was said to understand the message. Each step is complex, and many unanswered questions remain about how we communicate using language.

The brain controls all the complex events required to speak and understand language. That's why damage to the brain—such as that caused by interrupted blood flow during a stroke—can interfere with the ability to carry out these steps normally. Depending on where and how severely the brain is damaged, different problems can occur. These can be very severe (resulting in almost total inability to communicate) or relatively mild.

Because so many different things can be disturbed by damage to the brain, it's important for an aphasic person to have a thorough speech and language evaluation. To test the extent of the problems, a speech-language pathologist (sometimes called a speech therapist) must find out how well an aphasic person can speak and understand. A complete evaluation includes testing: verbal expression (speaking aloud); writing; understanding speech; and reading.

For some people, the language problems will be similar in all four areas. For others, some areas may have been spared and will continue to function normally. For example, sometimes reading and writing will be much harder than speaking. The different types of aphasia have many different names, but there's no set of "types" that everyone agrees upon. It's enough to know that aphasia can take different forms.

Aphasic people have trouble using language, but as a rule that doesn't mean they can't "think" clearly. Most aphasics know what they want to say; they just have trouble putting their thoughts into words. Some are unable to use "content" words, such as nouns or verbs, while others have trouble with "little" words like "the" and "of."

Some aphasic people speak very easily, even excessively, while others struggle to produce a sound. Sometimes people with aphasia are acutely aware of their problems; others don't seem to know they're hard to understand. Each person is different in the exact pattern of his or her language impairment.

The next section will help you find out which parts of communication are the most difficult for the aphasic person you know.

_____What You Can Do_____

While the Aphasic Patient Is in the Hospital

When you first see an aphasic patient in the hospital, you may be shocked or frightened. It may be especially disturbing if the person is in an intensive care unit. It's not easy to see a friend or loved one so critically ill, with tubes and wires everywhere. You may feel scared, faint or just uncomfortable. This is normal. Keep your first visits short, but keep coming back. You *will* get used to it.

People who've had a stroke are often cared for by a neurologist. That's the name for a doctor who specializes in diseases of the brain and other parts of the nervous system. The neurologist can explain the wires and tubes, and tell you about the patient's medical treatment. Clearly understanding the care being given will reassure you, and your explanations will, in turn, help reassure the patient.

Comforting and communicating with the patient will be most successful if you understand "your" patient's aphasia. A speech/language pathologist (speech therapist) is often the person best qualified to explain the problems to you. Many hospitals have a speech therapist on staff. Ask the neurologist or other doctor about this, and ask that the patient be seen as soon as possible.

After the patient has been tested, the speech therapist should meet with you and explain the person's communication strengths and weaknesses. The therapist should also give you a list of "do's" and "don'ts" to make communication easier. If the patient can begin speech/language therapy in the hospital, the speech therapist will tell you about progress.

Some hospitals don't have a speech/language pathologist on staff. If yours doesn't, or if there's a waiting list for services, ask the neurologist or other doctor to explain the type and severity of the person's aphasia. The nursing staff may also have useful information to share with you, since the nurses communicate with the patient regularly.

Although every patient is different, you can use some general guidelines to see how well the aphasic person can communicate.

Watch the person carefully while you ask short questions and make short requests. Can he or she respond correctly to your words alone? Or must you add gestures, like pointing to something, before the person can respond? Now make your questions and requests longer, and watch again.

Also, compare responses to conversations about immediate concerns (like the day's menu) and more remote topics (like politics). Now compare the responses when you talk rapidly in long sentences to those when you speak more slowly and in short phrases. It's important to watch the person's overall behavior very carefully, so you won't be misled.

Some patients, for example, smile and nod "yes" to almost every question. You may assume they understand perfectly, but in truth they may understand only a few key words. Other possibilities are that they're using only your gestures to understand what you mean, or guessing what you mean based on what normally happens during a familiar activity.

Remember, an aphasic person has probably not lost intelligence or common sense. Instead, he or she has lost some understanding and use of language. Once you know what kind of help a person needs, then always *give* that help. Don't spend your visits testing the person.

You can also get an idea of how well a patient can *say* what he or she wants to say. Can the person ask for things with a normal question? Or does he or she merely point or use single words? Are the words the right ones? Are real words mixed with made-up ones? Can the person carry on a superficial conversation but not say anything specific?

Again, watch carefully and give whatever help is needed.

After that, relax and let the person know that you'll try to understand all attempts to communicate.

Also, remember that aphasic people often have even *more* trouble reading and writing than in understanding and using *spoken* words. Therefore, writing down messages and asking them to respond by writing probably isn't a good idea. You may want to help by reading menu choices. Let the person watch while you read; you'll quickly find out whether he or she can read well enough to handle this alone.

Another way to help people with aphasia is to bring them their glasses, hearing aid and batteries, and dentures and dental adhesive (if needed). The occupational or physical therapist may also ask you to bring in some loose-fitting clothes and other personal items (e.g., electric razor).

Aphasic patients also may appreciate photos of friends, family members or events (such as a grandchild's birthday party) that occurred while they were in the hospital. Write the names and relationships of the people in the photos on the back. This will help the hospital staff and other visitors carry on interesting conversations. Patients may also enjoy tape-recorded messages from friends who can't visit in person.

Sample card for the aphasic person to carry:*

> *I have had a stroke, and it*
> *is hard for me to speak, read*
> *and write.*
> I usually understand what is said,
> but it helps if you speak clearly.
> Your help and patience would
> be appreciated. Thank You.

As an aphasic person begins to do more things alone, communication difficulties may lead to some unexpected and unfortunate situations. For example, slurred or slowed speech may *appear* to be the effect of drinking alcohol. If the patient is lost or needs information but can't clearly ask for help, others may think that he or she is "senile." In such cases, difficulties with speech and language caused by a stroke may give the *appearance* of being something entirely different.

*Provided by the American Heart Association.

It's a good idea for an aphasic person to carry some written identification and an explanation of the speech and language problems that the stroke caused. A card, such as the one in the middle of this booklet, may be useful. It's a good idea for aphasic people to carry a card that gives their address, phone number and perhaps destination, too.

Both in the home and the community, remember to approach the goal of independence slowly and realistically. And always keep safety in mind.

Resources

Here's a list of organizations you may want to contact for more information:

American Heart Association
(Look up your local or state chapter in the White Pages of your telephone book.)

American Occupational Therapy Association—national organization of occupational therapists.
American Occupational Therapy Association
1383 Piccard Drive
P.O. Box 1725
Rockville, MD 20849-1725
301-948-9626

American Physical Therapy Association—national organization of physical therapists.
American Physical Therapy Association
1111 N. Fairfax Street
Alexandria, VA 22314
703-684-2782

American Speech-Language-Hearing Association—national organization of speech/language pathologists and audiologists.
American Speech-Language-Hearing Association
10801 Rockville Pike
Rockville, MD 20852
Consumer Helpline—1-800-638-8255
In Maryland—1-301-897-8682 (Voice/TDD)

National Aphasia Association—national organization formed to help with the long-term needs of aphasic people and their families by giving them information and support.

National Aphasia Association
P.O. Box 1887
Murray Hill Station
New York, NY 10156-0611
212-263-6025

Stroke Clubs—local groups where people recovering from stroke and their families can meet, socialize, and gain support and information from others who've had a stroke or have had experience with someone who has.

V. Monica Pestrong
Easter Seal Society of
San Mateo County
1764 Marco Polo Way
Burlingame, CA 94010

Easter Seal Society of
Contra Costa/Solano/
Napa Counties
1303 Jefferson Street,
Suite #110A
Napa, CA 94558

Rosellen Sorenson
Easter Seal Society of
Alameda County
2757 Telegraph Avenue
Oakland, CA 94612

Easter Seal Society of
San Joaquin
102 West Bianchi Road
Stockton, CA 95207

Easter Seal Society of
Humboldt County
P.O. Box 109
3289 Edgewood (95501)
Eureka, CA 95502

Eugene Easter Seal
Service Center
3575 Donald Street
Eugene, OR 97405

Central Oregon Easter
Seal Society
51 N.W. Oregon Avenue
Bend, OR 97701

Todd Lowther
Colorado Easter Seal
Society
5755 West Alameda
Avenue
Lakewood, CO 80226

Easter Seal Society of
Utah
254 West 400 South
Suite 340
Salt Lake City, UT
84101

Pat Caldwell
Easter Seal Society of
Arizona
903 North Second Street
Phoenix, AZ 85004

Pat Caldwell
Easter Seal Society of
Yuma
P.O. Box 4966
2450 South Avenue A
Yuma, AZ 85364

Pat Caldwell
Easter Seal Society of
Tucson
5740 East 22nd Street
Tucson, AZ 85711

Michael Taylor
Easter Seal Society of
New Mexico
2819 Richmond Drive,
N.E.
Albuquerque, NM 87107

Vanessa Hunter
Easter Seal Thompson
House
1601 Ottawa Street
Joliet, IL 60432

Thomas King
North Texas Easter Seal
Rehabilitation
1005 Midwestern
Parkway E.
Wichita Falls, TX
76302-2211

Dona DeOtte
Brazos Valley
Rehabilitation Center
1318 Memorial Drive
Bryan, TX 77802

Lou Mangold
Easter Seal
Rehabilitation Center
2203 Babcock Road
San Antonio, TX 78229

Easter Seal Society
620 North Allegheny
Odessa, TX 79761

Maxine Kinsella
Easter Seal Society—
Program Site
1440 N.W. 15th Avenue
Aberdeen, SD 57401

Maxine Kinsella
Easter Seal Society of
South Dakota
115 East Sioux Avenue
Pierre, SD 57501

Maxine Kinsella
Easter Seal Society—
Program Site
Suite B5
2040 West Main
Rapid City, SD 57701

Maxine Kinsella
Easter Seal Society—
Program Site
430 Oriole Drive
Spearfish, SD 57783

Maxine Kinsella
Easter Seal Society of
South Dakota
c/o 2nd Edition
509 Main Avenue
Brookings, SD 57006

Maxine Kinsella
Easter Seal Society—
Program Site
R.R. 2, Box 33
La Bolt, SD 57246

Maxine Kinsella
Mitchell Easter Seal
Society
c/o St. Joseph Hospital
5th and Foster
Mitchell, SD 57301

Donna Jones
Easter Seal Society
708 Washington Street
P.O. Box 326
Woodstock, IL 60098

Cheryl Friebus
Jayne Shover Easter
Seal
P.O. Box 883
799 South McLean
Boulevard
Elgin, IL 60121

Victoria Proffat
Central Indiana Easter
Seal Society
Crossroads
Rehabilitation Center
4740 Kingsway Drive
Indianapolis, IN 46205

Gail Christ
The Easter Seal Center
2920 30th Street
Des Moines, IA 50310

Easter Seal
Rehabilitation Center,
Inc.
910 Myers Park Drive
Tallahassee, FL 32301

Easter Seal Center, Inc.
3661 South Babcock
Street
Melbourne, FL
32901-8221

Northern Kentucky
Easter Seal Center
212 Levassor Avenue
Covington, KY 41014

Mary Biel
Easter Seal
Rehabilitation Center
565 Children's Drive
West, P.O. Box 7166
Columbus, OH 43205

Easter Seal Center
231 Clark Road
Reading, OH 45215

Judith Jingst
Virginia Easter Seal
Center
P.O. Box 9185
3101 Magic Hollow
Boulevard 23456
Virginia Beach, VA
23450-9185

Virginia Easter Seal
Center
4841 Williamson Road
P.O. Box 5496
Roanoke, VA 24012

Richmond Areawide
Regional Office
6200 Chamberlayne
Road
Mechanicsville, VA
23111

Luanne K. Welch
Easter Seal Society
2315 Myron Drive
Raleigh, NC 27607

Jerry W. Mewbourn
Easter Seal Society of
South Carolina
3020 Farrow Road
Columbia, SC 23203

Easter Seal Society of
Greenville County
P.O. Box 8882
Station A
Greenville, SC 29605

Charles Webb Easter
Seal Center
325 Calhoun Street
Charleston, SC 29401

Waynesboro Treatment
Center
34 Roadside Avenue
Waynesboro, PA 17268

Mary Lou Steppling
Easter Seal Society of
Hazelton Area
301 Rocky Road and
Poplar Street
Hazelton, PA 18201

Ann Marie Liberty
Easter Seal Society
R.D. 2, Box 14
Blakely, PA 18447

Sheila Mehring
Easter Seal Society of
Maryland
3700 Fourth Street
Baltimore, MD 21225

Easter Seal Society
P.O. Box 231
Route 322 East
Franklin, PA 16323

Easter Seal Society of
Blair/Bedford
P.O. Box 1749
Altoona, PA 16603-1749

Easter Seal Society of
Franklin
55 Hamilton Avenue
Chambersburg, PA
17201

Easter Seal Camp
Fairlee Manor
Route 2, Box 319
Chestertown, MD 21620

Debra Nemchek
Easter Seal
Rehabilitation Center
26 Palmer's Hill Road
Stamford, CT 06902

Bonnie Graham
Easter Seal
Rehabilitation Center
22 Tompkins Street
Waterbury, CT 06708

Kristine Phillips
Easter Seal Society of
Monroe
9 Tobey Village Office
Park
Pittsford, NY 14534

Janet Bamberg
Massachusetts Easter
Seal Society
Denholm Building
484 Main Street, 6th
Floor
Worcester, MA 01608

Carol Fryer
Easter Seal Early
Intervention Program
44 Birch Street
Derry, NH 03038

Paul Boynton
Easter Seal Society of
New Hampshire
555 Auburn Street
Manchester, NH 03103

Ann Smith
Easter Seal Society
Brock Home
New Hampshire Easter
Seal Society
44 Fairview Street
Pittsfield, NH 03263

Easter Seal Society of
Maine
P.O. Box 518
84 Front Street
Bath, ME 04530

Hilo Service Center
P.O. Box 715
49 Kaiulani Street
Hilo, HI 96720

Easter Seal Society of
Alaska
3719 Arctic Boulevard
Anchorage, AK 99503

Additional information about strokes clubs is also available
from:
    National Easter Seal Society
    70 East Lake Street
    Chicago, IL 60601
    1-800/221-6827

    Your local chapter of the American Heart Association

Information may also be obtained from:
    National Stroke Association
    300 East Hampden Avenue
    Suite 240
    Englewood, CO 80110-2662

Last but not least, the organization with which I am
associated:
    The Stroke Foundation, Inc.
    898 Park Avenue
    New York, NY 10021
    212-734-3461

Vocational Rehabilitation Agency—local or state agency that
provides employment training for persons disabled by illness
or injury.

Contents of Foodstuffs

MEATS: FAT AND CHOLESTEROL COMPARISON CHART

Product (3½ oz, cooked)*	Saturated Fatty Acids (g)	Cholesterol (mg)	Total Fat[1] (g)	Calories from Fat[2] (%)	Total Calories
Beef					
Kidneys, simmered[3]	1.1	387	3.4	21	144
Liver, braised[3]	1.9	389	4.9	27	161
Round, top round, lean only, broiled	2.2	84	6.2	29	191

*3½ oz = 100 g (approximately).

[1] Total fat = saturated fatty acids plus monounsaturated fatty acids plus polyunsaturated fatty acids.

[2] Percent calories from fat = (total fat calories divided by total calories) multiplied by 100; total fat calories = total fat (grams) multiplied by 9.

[3] Liver and most organ meats are low in fat, but high in cholesterol. If you are eating to lower your blood cholesterol, you should consider your total cholesterol intake before selecting an organ meat.

— = Information not available in the sources used.

tr. = trace

Product (3½ oz, cooked)*	Saturated Fatty Acids (g)	Cholesterol (mg)	Total Fat[1] (g)	Calories from Fat[2] (%)	Total Calories
Round, eye of round, lean only, roasted	2.5	69	6.5	32	183
Round, tip round, lean only, roasted	2.8	81	7.5	36	190
Round, full cut, lean only, choice, broiled	2.9	82	8.0	37	194
Round, bottom round, lean only, braised	3.4	96	9.7	39	222
Short loin, top loin, lean only, broiled	3.6	76	8.9	40	203
Wedge-bone sirloin, lean only, broiled	3.6	89	8.7	38	208
Short loin, tenderloin, lean only, broiled	3.6	84	9.3	41	204
Chuck, arm pot roast, lean only, braised	3.8	101	10.0	39	231
Short loin, T-bone steak, lean only, choice, broiled	4.2	80	10.4	44	214

*3½ oz = 100 g (approximately).
[1] Total fat = saturated fatty acids plus monounsaturated fatty acids plus polyunsaturated fatty acids.
[2] Percent calories from fat = (total fat calories divided by total calories) multiplied by 100; total fat calories = total fat (grams) multiplied by 9.
[3] Liver and most organ meats are low in fat, but high in cholesterol. If you are eating to lower your blood cholesterol, you should consider your total cholesterol intake before selecting an organ meat.
— = Information not available in the sources used.
tr. = trace

Product (3½ oz, cooked)*	Saturated Fatty Acids (g)	Cholesterol (mg)	Total Fat[1] (g)	Calories from Fat[2] (%)	Total Calories
Short loin, porterhouse steak, lean only, choice, broiled	4.3	80	10.8	45	218
Brisket, whole, lean only, braised	4.6	93	12.8	48	241
Rib eye, small end (ribs 10–12), lean only, choice, broiled	4.9	80	11.6	47	225
Rib, whole (ribs 6–12), lean only, roasted	5.8	81	13.8	52	240
Flank, lean only, choice, braised	5.9	71	13.8	51	244
Rib, large end (ribs 6–9), lean only, broiled	6.1	82	14.2	55	233
Chuck, blade roast, lean only, braised	6.2	106	15.3	51	270
Corned beef, cured, brisket, cooked	6.3	98	19.0	68	251
Flank, lean and fat, choice, braised	6.6	72	15.5	54	257

*3½ oz = 100 g (approximately).

[1] Total fat = saturated fatty acids plus monounsaturated fatty acids plus polyunsaturated fatty acids.

[2] Percent calories from fat = (total fat calories divided by total calories) multiplied by 100; total fat calories = total fat (grams) multiplied by 9.

[3] Liver and most organ meats are low in fat, but high in cholesterol. If you are eating to lower your blood cholesterol, you should consider your total cholesterol intake before selecting an organ meat.

— = Information not available in the sources used.

tr. = trace

Product (3½ oz, cooked)*	Saturated Fatty Acids (g)	Cholesterol (mg)	Total Fat[1] (g)	Calories from Fat[2] (%)	Total Calories
Ground, lean, broiled medium	7.2	87	18.5	61	272
Round, full cut, lean and fat, choice, braised	7.3	84	18.2	60	274
Rib, short ribs, lean only, choice, braised	7.7	93	18.1	55	295
Salami, cured, cooked, smoked, 3–4 slices	9.0	65	20.7	71	262
Short loin, T-bone steak, lean and fat, choice, broiled	10.2	84	24.6	68	324
Chuck, arm pot roast, lean and fat, braised	10.7	99	26.0	67	350
Sausage, cured, cooked, smoked, about 2	11.4	67	26.9	78	312
Bologna, cured, 3–4 slices	12.1	58	28.5	82	312
Frankfurter, cured, about 2	12.0	61	28.5	82	315
Lamb					
Leg, lean only, roasted	3.0	89	8.2	39	191

*3½ oz = 100 g (approximately).

[1] Total fat = saturated fatty acids plus monounsaturated fatty acids plus polyunsaturated fatty acids.

[2] Percent calories from fat = (total fat calories divided by total calories) multiplied by 100; total fat calories = total fat (grams) multiplied by 9.

[3] Liver and most organ meats are low in fat, but high in cholesterol. If you are eating to lower your blood cholesterol, you should consider your total cholesterol intake before selecting an organ meat.

— = Information not available in the sources used.

tr. = trace

Product (3½ oz, cooked)*	Saturated Fatty Acids (g)	Cholesterol (mg)	Total Fat[1] (g)	Calories from Fat[2] (%)	Total Calories
Loin chop, lean only, broiled	4.1	94	9.4	39	215
Rib, lean only, roasted	5.7	88	12.3	48	232
Arm chop, lean only, braised	6.0	122	14.6	47	279
Rib, lean and fat, roasted	14.2	90	30.6	75	368
Pork					
Cured, ham steak, boneless, extra lean, unheated	1.4	45	4.2	31	122
Liver, braised[3]	1.4	355	4.4	24	165
Kidneys, braised[3]	1.5	480	4.7	28	151
Fresh, loin, tenderloin, lean only, roasted	1.7	93	4.8	26	166
Cured, shoulder, arm picnic, lean only, roasted	2.4	48	7.0	37	170
Cured, ham, boneless, regular, roasted	3.1	59	9.0	46	178
Fresh, leg (ham), shank half, lean only, roasted	3.6	92	10.5	44	215

*3½ oz = 100 g (approximately).

[1] Total fat = saturated fatty acids plus monounsaturated fatty acids plus polyunsaturated fatty acids.

[2] Percent calories from fat = (total fat calories divided by total calories) multiplied by 100; total fat calories = total fat (grams) multiplied by 9.

[3] Liver and most organ meats are low in fat, but high in cholesterol. If you are eating to lower your blood cholesterol, you should consider your total cholesterol intake before selecting an organ meat.

— = Information not available in the sources used.

tr. = trace

Product (3½ oz, cooked)*	Saturated Fatty Acids (g)	Cholesterol (mg)	Total Fat[1] (g)	Calories from Fat[2] (%)	Total Calories
Fresh, leg (ham), rump half, lean only, roasted	3.7	96	10.7	43	221
Fresh, loin, center loin, sirloin, lean only, roasted	4.5	91	13.1	49	240
Fresh, loin, sirloin, lean only, roasted	4.5	90	13.2	50	236
Fresh, loin, center rib, lean only, roasted	4.8	79	13.8	51	245
Fresh, loin, top loin, lean only, roasted	4.8	79	13.8	51	245
Fresh, shoulder, blade, Boston, lean only, roasted	5.8	98	16.8	59	256
Fresh, loin, blade, lean only, roasted	6.6	89	19.3	62	279
Fresh, loin, sirloin, lean and fat, roasted	7.4	91	20.4	63	291
Cured, shoulder, arm picnic, lean and fat, roasted	7.7	58	21.4	69	280

*3½ oz = 100 g (approximately).

[1] Total fat = saturated fatty acids plus monounsaturated fatty acids plus polyunsaturated fatty acids.

[2] Percent calories from fat = (total fat calories divided by total calories) multiplied by 100; total fat calories = total fat (grams) multiplied by 9.

[3] Liver and most organ meats are low in fat, but high in cholesterol. If you are eating to lower your blood cholesterol, you should consider your total cholesterol intake before selecting an organ meat.

— = Information not available in the sources used.

tr. = trace

Product	Saturated Fatty Acids (g)	Cholesterol (mg)	Total Fat[1] (g)	Calories from Fat[2] (%)	Total Calories
Fresh, loin, center loin, lean and fat, roasted	7.9	91	21.8	64	305
Cured, shoulder, blade roll, lean and fat, roasted	8.4	67	23.5	74	287
Fresh, Italian sausage, cooked	9.0	78	25.7	72	323
Fresh, bratwurst, cooked	9.3	60	25.9	77	301
Fresh, chitterlings, cooked	10.1	143	28.8	86	303
Cured, liver sausage, liverwurst	10.6	158	28.5	79	326
Cured, smoked link sausage, grilled	11.3	68	31.8	74	389
Fresh, spareribs, lean and fat, braised	11.8	121	30.3	69	397
Cured, salami, dry or hard	11.9	—	33.7	75	407
Bacon, fried	17.4	85	49.2	78	576

*3½ oz = 100 g (approximately).

[1] Total fat = saturated fatty acids plus monounsaturated fatty acids plus polyunsaturated fatty acids.

[2] Percent calories from fat = (total fat calories divided by total calories) multiplied by 100; total fat calories = total fat (grams) multiplied by 9.

[3] Liver and most organ meats are low in fat, but high in cholesterol. If you are eating to lower your blood cholesterol, you should consider your total cholesterol intake before selecting an organ meat.

— = Information not available in the sources used.

tr. = trace

Product (3½ oz, cooked)*	Saturated Fatty Acids (g)	Cholesterol (mg)	Total Fat[1] (g)	Calories from Fat[2] (%)	Total Calories
Veal					
Rump, lean only, roasted	—	128	2.2	13	156
Sirloin, lean only, roasted	—	128	3.2	19	153
Arm steak, lean only, cooked	—	90	5.3	24	200
Loin chop, lean only, cooked	—	90	6.7	29	207
Blade, lean only, cooked	—	90	7.8	33	211
Cutlet, medium fat, braised or broiled	4.8	128	11.0	37	271
Foreshank, medium fat, stewed	—	90	10.4	43	216
Plate, medium fat, stewed	—	90	21.2	63	303
Rib, medium fat, roasted	7.1	128	16.9	70	218
Flank, medium fat, stewed	—	90	32.3	75	390

SOURCES:

Composition of Foods: Beef Products—Raw • Processed • Prepared, Agriculture Handbook 8-13. United States Department of Agriculture, Human Nutrition Information Service (August 1986).

Composition of Foods: Pork Products—Raw • Processed • Prepared, Agriculture Handbook 8-10. United States Department of Agriculture, Human Nutrition Information Service (August 1983).

Home and Garden Bulletin. Nutritive Value of Foods. No. 72. United States Department of Agriculture, Human Nutrition Information Service (1986).

*3½ oz = 100 g (approximately).

[1] Total fat = saturated fatty acids plus monounsaturated fatty acids plus polyunsaturated fatty acids.

[2] Percent calories from fat = (total fat calories divided by total calories) multiplied by 100; total fat calories = total fat (grams) multiplied by 9.

[3] Liver and most organ meats are low in fat, but high in cholesterol. If you are eating to lower your blood cholesterol, you should consider your total cholesterol intake before selecting an organ meat.

— = Information not available in the sources used.

tr. = trace

POULTRY: FAT AND CHOLESTEROL COMPARISON CHART

Product (3½ oz, cooked)*	Saturated Fatty Acids (g)	Cholesterol (mg)	Total Fat[1] (g)	Calories from Fat[2] (%)	Total Calories
Turkey, fryer-roasters, light meat without skin, roasted	0.4	86	1.9	8	140
Chicken, roasters, light meat without skin, roasted	1.1	75	4.1	24	153
Turkey, fryer-roasters, light meat with skin, roasted	1.3	95	4.6	25	164
Chicken, broilers or fryers, light meat without skin, roasted	1.3	85	4.5	24	173
Turkey, fryer-roasters, dark meat without skin, roasted	1.4	112	4.3	24	162
Chicken, stewing, light meat without skin, stewed	2.0	70	8.0	34	213
Turkey roll, light and dark	2.0	55	7.0	42	149
Turkey, fryer-roasters, dark meat with skin, roasted	2.1	117	7.1	35	182
Chicken, roasters, dark meat without skin, roasted	2.4	75	8.8	44	178

Product (3½ oz, cooked)*	Saturated Fatty Acids (g)	Cholesterol (mg)	Total Fat[1] (g)	Calories from Fat[2] (%)	Total Calories
Chicken, broilers or fryers, dark meat without skin, roasted	2.7	93	9.7	43	205
Chicken, broilers or fryers, light meat with skin, roasted	3.0	85	10.9	44	222
Chicken, stewing, dark meat without skin, stewed	4.1	95	15.3	53	258
Duck, domesticated, flesh only, roasted	4.2	89	11.2	50	201
Chicken, broilers or fryers, dark meat with skin, roasted	4.4	91	15.8	56	253
Goose, domesticated, flesh only, roasted	4.6	96	12.7	48	238
Turkey bologna, about 3½ slices	5.1	99	15.2	69	199
Chicken frankfurter, about 2	5.5	101	19.5	68	257
Turkey frankfurter, about 2	5.9	107	17.7	70	226

SOURCE:
Composition of Foods: Poultry Products—Raw • Processed • Prepared, Agriculture Handbook 8-5.
United States Department of Agriculture, Science and Education Administration (August 1979).

FISH AND SHELLFISH:
FAT AND CHOLESTEROL COMPARISON CHART

Product (3½ oz, cooked)*	Saturated Fatty Acids (g)	Cholesterol (mg)	Omega-3 Fatty Acids (g)	Total Fat[1] (g)	Calories from Fat[2] (%)	Total Calories
Finfish						
Haddock, dry heat	0.2	74	0.2	0.9	7	112
Cod, Atlantic, dry heat	0.2	55	0.2	0.9	7	105
Pollock, walleye, dry heat	0.2	96	1.5	1.1	9	113
Perch, mixed species, dry heat	0.2	42	0.3	1.2	9	117
Grouper, mixed species, dry heat	0.3	47	—	1.3	10	118
Whiting, mixed species, dry heat	0.3	84	0.9	1.7	13	115
Snapper, mixed species, dry heat	0.4	47	—	1.7	12	128
Halibut, Atlantic and Pacific, dry heat	0.4	41	0.6	2.9	19	140
Rockfish, Pacific, dry heat	0.5	44	0.5	2.0	15	121
Sea bass, mixed species, dry heat	0.7	53	—	2.5	19	124
Trout, rainbow, dry heat	0.8	73	0.9	4.3	26	151
Swordfish, dry heat	1.4	50	1.1	5.1	30	155
Tuna, bluefin, dry heat	1.6	49	—	6.3	31	184
Salmon, sockeye, dry heat	1.9	87	1.3	11.0	46	216
Anchovy, European, canned	2.2	—	2.1	9.7	42	210

Product (3½ oz, cooked)*	Saturated Fatty Acids (g)	Cholesterol (mg)	Omega-3 Fatty Acids (g)	Total Fat[1] (g)	Calories from Fat[2] (%)	Total Calories
Herring, Atlantic, dry heat	2.6	77	2.1	11.5	51	203
Eel, dry heat	3.0	161	0.7	15.0	57	236
Mackerel, Atlantic, dry heat	4.2	75	1.3	17.8	61	262
Pompano, Florida, dry heat	4.5	64	—	12.1	52	211
Crustaceans						
Lobster, northern	0.1	72	0.1	0.6	6	98
Crab, blue, moist heat	0.2	100	0.5	1.8	16	102
Shrimp, mixed species, moist heat	0.3	195	0.3	1.1	10	99
Mollusks						
Whelk, moist heat	0.1	130	—	0.8	3	275
Clam, mixed species, moist heat	0.2	67	0.3	2.0	12	148
Mussel, blue, moist heat	0.9	56	0.8	4.5	23	172
Oyster, Eastern, moist heat	1.3	109	1.0	5.0	33	137

SOURCE:
Composition of Foods: Finfish and Shellfish Products—Raw • Processed • Prepared, Agriculture Handbook 8-15. United States Department of Agriculture (in press).

DAIRY AND EGG PRODUCTS:
FAT AND CHOLESTEROL COMPARISON CHART

Product	Saturated Fat (g)	Cholesterol (mg)	Total Fat[1] (g)	Calories from Fat[2] (%)	Total Calories
Milk (8 oz)					
Skim milk	0.3	4	0.4	5	86
Buttermilk	1.3	9	2.2	20	99
Low-fat milk, 1% fat	1.6	10	2.6	23	102
Low-fat milk, 2% fat	2.9	18	4.7	35	121
Whole milk, 3.3% fat	5.1	33	8.2	49	150
Yogurt (4 oz)					
Plain yogurt, low fat	0.1	2	0.2	3	63
Plain yogurt	2.4	14	3.7	47	70
Cheese					
Cottage cheese, lowfat, 1% fat, 4 oz	0.7	5	1.2	13	82
Mozzarella, part-skim, 1 oz	2.9	16	4.5	56	72
Cottage cheese, creamed, 4 oz	3.2	17	5.1	39	117
Mozzarella, 1 oz	3.7	22	6.1	69	80
Sour cream, 1 oz	3.7	12	5.9	87	61
American processed cheese spread, pasteurized, 1 oz	3.8	16	6.0	66	82
Feta, 1 oz	4.2	25	6.0	72	75
Neufchâtel, 1 oz	4.2	22	6.6	81	74

Product	Saturated Fatty Acids (g)	Cholesterol (mg)	Total Fat[1] (g)	Calories from Fat[2] (%)	Total Calories
Camembert, 1 oz	4.3	20	6.9	73	85
American processed cheese food, pasteurized, 1 oz	4.4	18	7.0	68	93
Provolone, 1 oz	4.8	20	7.6	68	100
Limburger, 1 oz	4.8	26	7.7	75	93
Brie, 1 oz	4.9	28	7.9	74	95
Romano, 1 oz	4.9	29	7.6	63	110
Gouda, 1 oz	5.0	32	7.8	69	101
Swiss, 1 oz	5.0	26	7.8	65	107
Edam, 1 oz	5.0	25	7.9	70	101
Brick, 1 oz	5.3	27	8.4	72	105
Blue, 1 oz	5.3	21	8.2	73	100
Gruyere, 1 oz	5.4	31	9.2	71	117
Muenster, 1 oz	5.4	27	8.5	74	104
Parmesan, 1 oz	5.4	22	8.5	59	129
Monterey Jack, 1 oz	5.5	25	8.6	73	106
Roquefort, 1 oz	5.5	26	8.7	75	105
Ricotta, part-skim, 4 oz	5.6	25	9.0	52	156
American processed cheese, pasteurized, 1 oz	5.6	27	8.9	75	106
Colby, 1 oz	5.7	27	9.1	73	112
Cheddar, 1 oz	6.0	30	9.4	74	114

Product	Saturated Fatty Acids (g)	Cholesterol (mg)	Total Fat[1] (g)	Calories from Fat[2] (%)	Total Calories
Cream cheese, 1 oz	6.2	31	9.9	90	99
Ricotta, whole milk, 4 oz	9.4	58	14.7	67	197
Eggs					
Egg, chicken, white	0	0	tr.	0	16
Egg, chicken, whole	1.7	274	5.6	64	79
Egg, chicken, yolk	1.7	272	5.6	80	63

SOURCE:
Composition of Foods: Dairy and Egg Products—Raw • Processed • Prepared, Agriculture Handbook 8-1. United States Department of Agriculture, Agricultural Research Service (November 1976).

FATS AND OILS COMPARISON CHART

Product (1 Tbsp)	Saturated Fatty Acids (g)	Cholesterol (mg)	Poly-unsaturated Fatty Acids (g)	Mono-unsaturated Fatty Acids (g)
Rapeseed oil (canola oil)	0.9	0	4.5	7.6
Safflower oil	1.2	0	10.1	1.6
Sunflower oil	1.4	0	5.5	6.2
Peanut butter, smooth	1.5	0	2.3	3.7
Corn oil	1.7	0	8.0	3.3
Olive oil	1.8	0	1.1	9.9
Hydrogenated sunflower oil	1.8	0	4.9	6.3
Margarine, liquid, bottled	1.8	0	5.1	3.9
Margarine, soft, tub	1.8	0	3.9	4.8
Sesame oil	1.9	0	5.7	5.4
Soybean oil	2.0	0	7.9	3.2
Margarine, stick	2.1	0	3.6	5.1
Peanut oil	2.3	0	4.3	6.2
Cottonseed oil	3.5	0	7.1	2.4
Lard	5.0	12	1.4	5.8
Beef tallow	6.4	14	0.5	5.3
Palm oil	6.7	0	1.3	5.0
Butter	7.1	31	0.4	3.3
Cocoa butter	8.1	0	0.4	4.5
Palm kernel oil	11.1	0	0.2	1.5
Coconut oil	11.8	0	0.2	0.8

SOURCES:
Composition of Foods: Fats and Oils—Raw • Processed • Prepared, Agriculture Handbook 8-4. United States Department of Agriculture, Science and Education Administration (June 1979).

Composition of Foods: Legumes and Legume Products—Raw • Processed • Prepared, Agriculture Handbook 8-16. United States Department of Agriculture, Human Nutrition Information Service (December 1986).

NUTS AND SEEDS: FAT COMPARISON CHART

Product (1 oz)	Saturated Fatty Acids (g)	Cholesterol (mg)	Total Fat[1] (g)	Calories from Fat[2] (%)	Total Calories
European chestnuts	0.2	0	1.1	9	105
Filberts or hazelnuts	1.3	0	17.8	89	179
Almonds	1.4	0	15.0	80	167
Pecans	1.5	0	18.4	89	187
Sunflower seed kernels, roasted	1.5	0	1.4	77	165
English walnuts	1.6	0	17.6	87	182
Pistachio nuts	1.7	0	13.7	75	164
Peanuts	1.9	0	14.0	76	164
Hickory nuts	2.0	0	18.3	88	187
Pine nuts, pignolia	2.2	0	14.4	89	146
Pumpkin and squash seed kernels	2.3	0	12.0	73	148
Cashew nuts	2.6	0	13.2	73	163
Macadamia nuts	3.1	0	20.9	95	199
Brazil nuts	4.6	0	18.8	91	186
Coconut meat, unsweetened	16.3	0	18.3	88	187

SOURCES:
Composition of Foods: Legumes and Legume Products—Raw • Processed • Prepared, Agriculture Handbook 8–16. United States Department of Agriculture, Human Nutrition Information Service (December 1986).

Composition of Foods: Nut and Seed Products—Raw • Processed • Prepared, Agriculture Handbook 8-12. United States Department of Agriculture, Human Nutrition Information Service (September 1984).

BREADS, CEREALS, PASTA, RICE, AND DRIED PEAS AND BEANS:
FAT AND CHOLESTEROL COMPARISON CHART

Product	Saturated Fatty Acids (g)	Cholesterol (mg)	Total Fat[1] (g)	Calories from Fat[2] (%)	Total Calories
Breads					
Melba toast, 1 plain	0.1	0	tr.	0	20
Pita, ½ large shell	0.1	0	1.0	5	165
Corn tortilla	0.1	0	1.0	14	65
Rye bread, 1 slice	0.2	0	1.0	14	65
English muffin	0.3	0	1.0	6	140
Bagel, 1, 3½" diameter	0.3	0	2.0	9	200
White bread, 1 slice	0.3	0	1.0	14	65
RyKrisp, 2 triple crackers	0.3	0	1.0	16	56
Whole wheat bread, 1 slice	0.4	0	1.0	13	70
Saltines, 4	0.5	4	1.0	18	50
Hamburger bun	0.5	tr.	2.0	16	115
Hot dog bun	0.5	tr.	2.0	16	115
Pancake, 1, 4" diameter	0.5	16	2.0	30	60
Bran muffin, 1, 2½" diameter	1.4	24	6.0	43	125
Corn muffin, 1, 2½" diameter	1.5	23	5.0	31	145
Plain doughnut, 1, 3¼" diameter	2.8	20	12.0	51	210

Product	Saturated Fatty Acids (g)	Cholesterol (mg)	Total Fat[1] (g)	Calories from Fat[2] (%)	Total Calories
Croissant, 1, 4½″ by 4″	3.5	13	12.0	46	235
Waffle, 1, 7″ diameter	4.0	102	13.0	48	245
Cereals (1 cup)					
Corn flakes	tr.	—	0.1	0	98
Cream of Wheat, cooked	tr.	—	0.5	3	134
Corn grits, cooked	tr.	—	0.5	3	146
Oatmeal, cooked	0.4	—	2.4	15	145
Granola	5.8	—	33.1	50	595
100% Natural Cereal with raisins and dates	13.7	—	20.3	37	496
Pasta (1 cup)					
Spaghetti, cooked	0.1	0	1.0	6	155
Elbow macaroni, cooked	0.1	0	1.0	6	155
Egg noodles, cooked	0.5	50	2.0	11	160
Chow mein noodles, canned	2.1	5	11.0	45	220
Rice (1 cup cooked)					
Rice, white	0.1	0	0.5	2	225
Rice, brown	0.3	0	1.0	4	230

Product	Saturated Fatty Acids (g)	Cholesterol (mg)	Total Fat[1] (g)	Calories from Fat[2] (%)	Total Calories
Dried Peas and Beans (1 cup cooked)					
Split peas	0.1	0	0.8	3	231
Kidney beans	0.1	0	1.0	4	225
Lima beans	0.2	0	0.7	3	217
Black-eyed peas	0.3	0	1.2	5	200
Garbanzo beans	0.4	0	4.3	14	269

SOURCES:
Composition of Foods: Breakfast Cereals—Raw • Processed • Prepared, Agriculture Handbook 8-8. United States Department of Agriculture, Human Nutrition Service (July 1982).
Composition of Foods: Legumes and Legume Products—Raw • Processed • Prepared, Agriculture Handbook 8–16. United States Department of Agriculture, Human Nutrition Monitoring Division (December 1986).
Home and Garden Bulletin, Nutritive Value of Foods, No. 72. United States Department of Agriculture, Human Nutrition Information Service (1986).

SWEETS AND SNACKS:
FAT AND CHOLESTEROL COMPARISON CHART

Product	Saturated Fatty Acids (g)	Cholesterol (mg)	Total Fat[1] (g)	Calories from Fat[2] (%)	Total Calories
Beverages					
Ginger ale, 12 oz	0.0	0	0.0	0	125
Cola, regular, 12 oz	0.0	0	0.0	0	160
Chocolate shake, 10 oz	6.5	37	10.5	26	360
Candy (1 oz)					
Hard candy	0.0	0	0.0	0	110
Gum drops	tr.	0	tr.	tr.	100
Fudge	2.1	1	3.0	24	115
Milk chocolate, plain	5.4	6	9.0	56	145
Cookies					
Vanilla wafers, 5 cookies, 1¾" diameter	0.9	12	3.3	32	94
Fig bars, 4 cookies, 1⅝" by 1⅝" by ⅜"	1.0	27	4.0	17	210
Chocolate brownie with icing, 1½" by 1¾" by ⅞"	1.6	14	4.0	36	100
Oatmeal cookies, 4 cookies, 2⅝" diameter	2.5	2	10.0	37	245

Product	Saturated Fatty Acids (g)	Cholesterol (mg)	Total Fat[1] (g)	Calories from Fat[2] (%)	Total Calories
Chocolate chip cookies, 4 cookies, 2¼" diameter	3.9	18	11.0	54	185

Cakes and Pies

Product	Saturated Fatty Acids (g)	Cholesterol (mg)	Total Fat[1] (g)	Calories from Fat[2] (%)	Total Calories
Angel food cake, 1/12 of 10" cake	tr.	0	tr.	tr.	125
Gingerbread, 1/9 of 8" cake	1.1	1	4.0	21	175
White layer cake, with white icing, 1/16 of 9" cake	2.1	3	9.0	32	260
Yellow layer cake with chocolate icing, 1/16 of 9" cake	3.0	36	8.0	31	235
Pound cake, 1/17 of loaf	3.0	64	5.0	41	110
Devil's food cake with chocolate icing, 1/16 of 9" cake	3.5	37	8.0	31	235
Lemon meringue pie, 1/6 of 9" pie	4.3	143	14.0	36	355
Apple pie, 1/6 of 9" pie	4.6	0	18.0	40	405
Cream pie, 1/6 of 9" pie	15.0	8	23.0	46	455

Snacks

Product	Saturated Fatty Acids (g)	Cholesterol (mg)	Total Fat[1] (g)	Calories from Fat[2] (%)	Total Calories
Popcorn, air-popped, 1 cup	tr.	0	tr.	tr.	30

Product	Saturated Fatty Acids (g)	Cholesterol (mg)	Total Fat[1] (g)	Calories from Fat[2] (%)	Total Calories
Pretzels, stick, 2¼", 10 pretzels	tr.	0	tr.	tr.	10
Popcorn with oil and salted, 1 cup	0.5	0	3.0	49	55
Corn chips, 1 oz	1.4	25	9.0	52	155
Potato chips, 1 oz	2.6	0	10.1	62	147
Pudding					
Gelatin	0.0	0	0.0	0	70
Tapioca, ½ cup	2.3	15	4.0	25	145
Chocolate pudding, ½ cup	2.4	15	4.0	24	150

SOURCE:
Home and Garden Bulletin, Nutritive Value of Foods. No. 72. United States Department of Agriculture, Human Nutrition Information Service (1986).

MISCELLANEOUS:
FAT AND CHOLESTEROL COMPARISON CHART

Product	Saturated Fatty Acids (g)	Cholesterol (mg)	Total Fat[1] (g)	Calories from Fat[2] (%)	Total Calories
Gravies (½ cup)					
Au jus, canned	0.1	1	0.3	3	80
Turkey, canned	0.7	3	2.5	37	61
Beef, canned	1.4	4	2.8	41	62
Chicken, canned	1.7	3	6.8	65	95
Sauces (½ cup)					
Sweet and sour	tr.	0	0.1	<1	147
Barbecue	0.3	0	2.3	22	94
White	3.2	17	6.7	50	121
Cheese	4.7	26	8.6	50	154
Sour cream	8.5	45	15.1	53	255
Hollandaise	20.9	94	34.1	87	353
Bearnaise	20.9	99	34.1	88	351
Salad Dressings (1 Tbsp)					
Russian, low calorie	0.1	1	0.7	27	23
French, low calorie	0.1	1	0.9	37	22
Italian, low calorie	0.2	1	1.5	85	16
Thousand Island, low calorie	0.2	2	1.6	59	24
Imitation mayonnaise	0.5	4	2.9	75	35
Thousand Island, regular	0.9	—	5.6	86	59
Italian, regular	1.0	—	7.1	93	69
Russian, regular	1.1	—	7.8	92	76
French, regular	1.5	—	6.4	86	67

Product	Saturated Fatty Acids (g)	Cholesterol (mg)	Total Fat[1] (g)	Calories from Fat[2] (%)	Total Calories
Blue cheese	1.5	—	8.0	93	77
Mayonnaise	1.6	8	11.0	100	99
Other					
Olives, green, 4 medium	0.2	0	1.5	90	15
Nondairy creamer, powdered, 1 teaspoon	0.7	0	1.0	90	10
Avocado, Florida	5.3	0	27.0	72	340
Pizza, cheese, ⅛ of 15″ diameter	4.1	56	9.0	28	290
Quiche lorraine, ⅛ of 8″ diameter	23.2	285	48.0	72	600

SOURCES:
Composition of Foods: Fats and Oils—Raw • Processed • Prepared, Agriculture Handbook 8-4. United States Department of Agriculture, Science and Education Administration (June 1979).

Composition of Foods: Soups, Sauces, and Gravies—Raw • Processed • Prepared, Agriculture Handbook 8-6. United States Department of Agriculture, Science and Education Administration (February 1980).

Home and Garden Bulletin, Nutritive Value of Foods. No. 72. United States Department of Agriculture, Human Nutrition Information Service (1986).

Glossary

ACE inhibitors (angiotensin converting enzyme inhibitors). Medications that inhibit the action of angiotensin and thereby lower blood pressure.

Adrenal gland. A small but powerful gland sitting on top of each kidney that produces hormones that can cause high blood pressure. Adrenalin (epinephrine) and aldosterone are examples of these hormones.

Amino acids. Building blocks of protein. Combinations of amino acids make a protein.

Anemia. A condition in which the number of red blood cells or the amount of hemoglobin is below normal. It can be caused by bleeding, iron deficiency, and other disorders.

Aneurysm. Localized weakness in the wall of an artery or vein may produce a bulge in the wall. The bulge is known as an aneurysm.

Angiogram. An X ray of the blood vessels and/or heart, performed by injecting dye into the bloodstream.

Angiotensin. A substance produced in the body that raises the blood pressure by constricting blood vessels.

Antihypertensives. Drugs used to lower blood pressure.

Aorta. The largest artery in the body. It receives blood from the heart and distributes it through the arteries to the entire body.

Aphasia. Inability to express oneself through words.

Apoplexy. See Cerebral hemorrhage.

Arteriosclerosis. A condition where there is thickening of the walls of the artery accompanied by loss of elasticity. (See also Atherosclerosis.)

Arteriovenous malformation. A tangle of arteries and veins.

Artery. The conduit (tube) carrying blood from the heart that supplies our tissues with oxygen and other nourishment.

Atherosclerosis. The buildup of fatty deposits (plaque) on the inner surface of arteries. A factor in Arteriosclerosis.

Beta blockers. Medication used to treat high blood pressure and angina. It works by blocking adrenalinelike substances.

Blood fat. Blood fats include cholesterol, triglycerides, and other substances. The fat generally associated with hardening of the arteries is cholesterol. Fats are normal constituents of the blood and are considered dangerous only when levels become excessive.

Blood pressure. The pressure in the arteries generated by the heart pumping blood. (See also Systolic blood pressure and Diastolic blood pressure.)

Bradycardia. An abnormally slow heart rate.

Brain infarction. A type of stroke caused by the death of brain tissue.

Bruit. A murmur of noise arising in a blood vessel, usually as a result of narrowing of the blood vessel.

Calcium channel blockers. Medication used in the treatment of hypertension, angina, and some heartbeat irregularities. They work by preventing calcium's effect on the smooth muscle in arteries. This reduces constriction of the arteries.

Carotid arteries. Chief arteries in the neck and head.

Cerebral hemorrhage. Bleeding within the brain as a result of blood vessels that burst, preventing flow of blood and damaging that part of the brain.

Cerebrovascular. Pertaining to the blood vessels of the brain.

Cholesterol. A fatty substance manufactured in the body and also obtained through our diet. Used for production of hormones and other processes. Implicated as a cause of heart attacks and strokes.

Circle of Willis. A "circle" at the base of the brain where the four principal arteries to the brain join before branching off to supply the brain with blood containing oxygen and glucose.

Computerized tomography (CT) scan. X-ray slices of tissue with computer coordination produces cross-sectional images of body tissues.

Congenital. Implies a condition that is present at birth.

Diabetes. A disorder of metabolism characterized by problems in the utilization of glucose.

Diastolic blood pressure. In a blood pressure of 120/80, the lower figure of 80 is the diastolic blood pressure.

Diuretics. Medication that increases the output of urine and the elimination of sodium from the body.

Electrocardiogram (EKG or ECG). A record of the heart's electrical action.

Embolic stroke. Stroke caused by clots, which may form on heart valves and travel to the brain.

Embolus.   A clot forming in one place, breaking off, and moving through the arteries to a distant place.

Endarterectomy.   Surgical procedure to remove fatty deposits that narrow an artery.

Epinephrine.   See Adrenal gland.

Essential hypertension.   Essential hypertension is synonymous with primary hypertension. In this form of high blood pressure, there is no known cause.

Estrogen.   The female hormone produced by the ovaries. No longer produced after menopause.

Hemiplegia.   Paralysis or weakness on one half of the body.

Hemorrhage.   Abnormal bleeding. In a brain hemorrhage, a blood vessel ruptures for any number of reasons, causing bleeding within the brain with consequent deprivation of that part of the brain of vital oxygen and glucose.

High density lipoprotein (HDL).   A protein that carries the good cholesterol in the blood. May be involved in the removal of excess cholesterol from the walls of the arteries.

Hyperlipidemia.   Excessive amount of fats in the blood.

Hypertension.   High blood pressure.

Hypoglycemia.   Low levels of blood glucose in the blood.

Infarction.   An area of tissue in an organ that has died. If the death of tissue is in the brain, the infarction is commonly called stroke. A myocardial infarction is death of heart tissue, commonly called a coronary or heart attack.

Intensive care unit.   A room especially designed to care for critically ill patients. All the body's vital signs (respiration, heart rate, blood pressure, and electrocardiogram) can be monitored through special electronic equipment.

Ischemia.   Low levels of oxygen in tissue because of obstruction in an artery.

Ischemic brain tissue.   Disease of the brain caused by a lack of oxygen. This is commonly caused by hardening of the arteries to the brain.

Ischemic heart disease. Disease of the heart caused by a lack of oxygen. This is commonly caused by hardening of the arteries to the heart.

Lanthanic disease. A disease without symptoms. Examples of lanthanic diseases are early diabetes, tuberculosis, hardening of the arteries, and high blood pressure.

Lesion. An injury or wound. An atherosclerotic lesion is an injury to an artery due to hardening of the arteries.

Lipoprotein. Literally fat-protein. Fat is hooked up to protein in the blood and is carried in the blood as lipoprotein. This, in effect, does for blood fat what homogenization does for milk fat. There are different types of lipoproteins: a very low density, low density, and high density lipoproteins. The density is measured by the size of the particles and different physical properties. Low density lipoproteins are the chief carriers of cholesterol.

Low density lipoprotein (LDL). The protein that carries the so-called bad cholesterol in the blood.

Magnetic resonance imaging (MRI). A noninvasive procedure utilizing a magnetic field, producing images of the body's organs.

Metabolism. The chemical and physical processes of life. Consists of catabolic (breakdown) and anabolic (building) processes.

Milligram. A thousandth of a gram (abbreviated mg.). A gram equals 1/30 of an ounce.

Monosaturated fat. Peanut and olive oil. These fats have little effect on cholesterol levels in the blood.

Myocardial infarction. A heart attack. See Infarction.

Noninvasive procedures. Do not involve instruments entering the body.

Obesity. Body weight about 20 percent or more than standards for age, height, and sex.

Orthostatic hypotension. Low blood pressure occurring after standing. May cause fainting.

Pacemaker. An artificial device placed in the heart that provides a desirable rate of heartbeat.

Pheochromocytoma. A tumor of the adrenal gland that causes high blood pressure.

Physiatry. The medical specialty devoted to rehabilitation.

Plaque. A stage of hardening of the arteries. Plaques are formed in the arteries as the result of deposits of fat and other components in the walls of the arteries. They partially obstruct the arteries and can lead to clot formation—thrombosis in the arteries.

Platelets. The smallest of the three types of cells in the blood. Important in clotting and other processes.

Polyunsaturated fat. These are the liquid vegetable fats, such as corn oil, safflower oil, walnut oil, cottonseed oil, and others (except coconut oil). They tend to act in such a way as to lower cholesterol in the blood.

Positron emission tomography (PET) scanning. Radioisotopic scanning used to study metabolic processes and blood flow.

Prudent diet. A diet low in cholesterol and saturated fats.

Red blood cells. One of the three types of cells in the blood, whose function is to carry hemoglobin that transports the oxygen.

Renal hypertension. High blood pressure secondary to kidney disease of different types. Glomerulonephritis and pyelonephritis are examples of kidney diseases that can cause high blood pressure.

Saturated fat. Basically, fats and oils of animal origin that tend to elevate blood fats and cholesterol. Coconut oil, while a vegetable oil, is the exception—it, too, is a saturated fat.

Secondary hypertension. High blood pressure resulting from diseases that can be identified, for example, kidney disease, tumors of the adrenal glands, and coarctation of the aorta.

Stenosis. The narrowing of an artery.

Stroke. Interference of blood supply to the brain, resulting in varying degrees of disability.

Subarachnoid hemorrhage. Bleeding in the area between two of the covering layers of the brain that contains the spinal fluid.

Syncope. Fainting.

Systolic blood pressure. In a blood pressure of 120/80, the upper number of 120 is the systolic blood pressure.

Thrombosis. Blockage or obstruction of an artery, resulting from a clot in the artery.

Thrombus. The clot blocking or obstructing the artery.

Tissue plasminogen activator (TPA). A clot-dissolving substance produced by the body and also produced by genetic engineering. Another clot dissolver is called streptokinase.

Transient ischemic attack (TIA or ministroke). Warning signs of a stroke: A temporary stroke, usually lasting for a few minutes. TIAs generally leave no permanent effects; between attacks, a person is completely normal.

Triglyceride. One of the fats found in blood and our fat stores in the body. It may play a role in arteriosclerosis.

Vasovagal response. An example would include people who faint at the sight of blood.

Vein. The conduit (tube) going to the heart, carrying blood containing carbon dioxide and waste products from the tissues.

Index